HIDDEN LIVES

Revised & Updated

Hidden LIVES

TRUE STORIES *from* **PEOPLE** *who* **LIVE** *with* **MENTAL ILLNESS**

Foreword by **GABOR MATÉ, MD**

Edited by **LENORE ROWNTREE**
& ANDREW BODEN

BRINDLE
& GLASS

First edition (with subtitle *Coming Out on Mental Illness*) published 2012.
Revised & updated edition published 2017.

Brindle & Glass, an imprint of TouchWood Editions
brindleandglass.com

LIBRARY AND ARCHIVES CANADA CATALOGUING IN PUBLICATION
Hidden lives : true stories from people who live with mental illness /
edited by Andrew Boden, Lenore Rowntree ; foreword by Gabor Maté.

Issued in print and electronic formats.
ISBN 978-1-927366-53-0

1. Mental illness. 2. Mentally ill Biography. I. Boden, Andrew, editor
II. Rowntree, Lenore, editor

RC464.A1H54 2017   362.196'8900922   C20179003941

Proofreader: Heather Sangster, Strong Finish
Design: Pete Kohut
Cover image: FreeImages.com/Kimberly Vohsen

We acknowledge the financial support of the Government of
Canada through the Canada Book Fund and the Canada Council
for the Arts, and of the province of British Columbia through the
British Columbia Arts Council and the Book Publishing Tax Credit.

 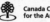

The interior pages of this book have been printed on 100% post-consumer
recycled paper, processed chlorine free, and printed with vegetable-based inks.

PRINTED IN CANADA AT FRIESENS

17 18 19 20 21   5 4 3 2 1

■ ■ ■

For those who have shown that
stigma and bias can be beaten

■ ■ ■

Contents

Foreword | GABOR MATÉ, MD | 1
Introduction | LENORE ROWNTREE | 3
Aftermath | FIONA TINWEI LAM | 7

Wellspring
Bad Day | JOEL YANOFSKY | 10
The Path to Sanity | JAMIE JOHNSON | 18
The Last Call | JILL SADOWSKY | 29
Stormtrooper | DELL CATHERALL | 37
Raising Julie | SARA DEMETER | 46

Into the Bell Jar
Elm | SHANE NEILSON | 56
Over and Overcoming | YAHO-HANAN FIWCHUK | 64
Atlas & the Cheese Cube | CATHERINE OWEN | 72
Bipolar Babe | ANDREA PAQUETTE | 80
Committed | ADDY S. PARKER | 84
Code Three | SCOTT WHYTE | 94
Crazy: One Woman's Search for Sanity | GAIL MARLENE SCHWARTZ | 103
Late Summer, Early Fall, as Told to the Dead of Winter | MEREDITH DARLING | 113
Life with My Mongrel | LYNNE VAN LUVEN | 122
The Biology of Human Starvation | LAURA INGRAM | 132
Rainy Day | CLARISSA HART | 138

My Brother, My Sister
In a Quiet Room | ANDREW BODEN | 148
On the Way to Here | JUDY McFARLANE | 159
Haunted | LAUREN McGUIRE | 165
Pennies in My Pocket: Stories of My Brother | LAURA TRUNKEY | 176
Only Love Taps | NICOLE MELCHIONDA | 186

Times Long Past
Covering for My Father | DOUGLAS TODD | 196
Lessons from Uncle Charles | JENNIFER CROWDER | 204
Hindsight | ERIN HART MacNAIR | 216
Flying Wounded | SUSAN McCASLIN | 221
Dislocated Tongues | KEVIN SPENST | 236
Belly Button | JANE FINLAY-YOUNG | 244

Family Constellation
One Girl in the Crowd | BETH ROWNTREE | 252
Flat Champagne | LENORE ROWNTREE | 260

Afterword | ANDREW BODEN | 267
Notes on Contributors | | 270

Foreword

GABOR MATÉ, MD

"If Doron's body were hurting, people would send gifts, but because it's his mind, they throw bricks." So writes a perceptive and anguished thirteen-year-old girl of her brother's mental illness in an early story of this brave and fascinating collection.

Hidden Lives is not about mental illness in the usual sense of the topic being studied, described, or analyzed. It is concerned with the very essence of psycho-emotional breakdown, refracted through the personal recollections of people directly touched by it, whether family members or sufferers. In a few highly illuminating cases, we are presented with depictions of the same episode of mental illness as experienced both by the individual and their close ones. We get a privileged if uncomfortably close look at one of the most devastating of human tribulations. Parents coming to terms with the autism diagnosis of a small child or the suicide of an adult one speak their heart's sorrow in these pages.

"As I treated these patients, I felt like I was wearing a rapidly fraying disguise," writes a medical doctor who only with the greatest effort can mask his own unravelling mental state as he cares for people in an Emergency Ward. That perceived need to cover up, to hide the self from the gaze of others and from the feared judgments and opprobrium of society, magnifies the torment endured by the sufferer. And this fear, even in our relatively enlightened age, after more than a century of modern psychiatric and psychological information being available to the public, is not paranoid. *Crazy, neurotic, retarded, psycho*—such words are still hurled about as insults. "The stigma associated with mental illness implies that people who have one are unintelligent," writes a young woman with bipolar disorder, a stigma reinforced not only by her own

1

self-beliefs but also by her friends and family. All too often, as we see in these stories, such negative self-images are reflected back to the sufferer in the incomprehension, lack of empathy, or lack of insight on the part of the health professionals charged with making the person better.

And worse. If a person had, say, heart disease, his or her capacity to make rational decisions would remain relatively unimpaired. A core dilemma of mental illness, as revealed in story after story in this book, is that the very organ of insight and thought—the brain—is the diseased entity. As the same physician writes, "The thing illness robs us of, mental illness most of all, is perspective: we never really apprehend how sick we are until it's either too late or until we get well again."

For all the raw honesty of its revelations, *Hidden Lives* communicates not despair but courage. We witness here the determination to struggle on in the face of invisible demons that have captured one's emotions and thoughts; the courage of family members whose lot it has become to live with and endure the mental dysfunction and agony, or even the death, of a loved one. This courage to be with and to accept the unthinkable is, ultimately, the greatest manifestation of our humanity.

Introduction

LENORE ROWNTREE

Sometimes the radio can be more than annoying. I was ten years old, standing in front of the bedroom mirror listening to the CBC, Canada's national broadcaster, on my turquoise transistor, when a grave-sounding social worker's voice came from the radio and riveted me to the spot. The voice said the incidence of child abuse goes up in homes where there are difficult children. There was a difficult child in our house. I wondered what this meant for us.

It wasn't abuse from my parents that frightened me; I knew there wasn't going to be any. What frightened me then, and still does, was the realization that I was too worn out to have children of my own. I'd already used up a lifetime of nurturing energy on my little sister, who suffered with childhood schizophrenia. I didn't know how to talk about this with anyone—it just seemed too crazy.

When I was older, I learned that even if I did figure out a way to talk about it, nobody wanted to hear. Not my girlfriends who straggled home from high school beside me, not my teachers—why are your marks so bad?—not even most of my relatives. My sister was in the same category as the aunt who'd divorced in disgrace— just don't talk about it, period.

The 1960s and 1970s were a confusing time for anyone trying to sort out psychiatric mysteries. On the one hand, it was a status symbol to be in psychoanalysis; on the other, the legislation in the country still described people in need of care and compassion as imbeciles and idiots. As a teenager, my solution to the problem was to read R.D. Laing and Thomas Szasz, both of whom claimed there was no such thing as mental illness. I realize now I was reading mostly to convince myself that my sister wasn't sick. This, of course, meant that I couldn't get sick either.

3

It took a long time for me to get over my own psychodrama and see that I was not at the centre of this issue. It was my sister's issue, a health issue that spelled tragedy for her, and one for which there was little support or sympathy. Some misinformed people see "mental illness" as an excuse for bad behaviour. And for a significant number, myself included, there is an element of fear, a mentalphobia. We're all a bit afraid it might happen to us, so why rub shoulders with it? Except that it's a part of life. Health Canada and the American NAMI (National Alliance on Mental Health) both estimate 20 per cent of us will experience a mental illness during our lifetime. If you add to this number all the family members of those affected, it means virtually every North American is or will be touched by the issue.

My co-editor, Andrew Boden, and I wanted to create this anthology to help lift the veil of mystery, to begin to remove the stigma, to normalize the issues around mental illness. We hope the illness can start to become just another part of life. When Andrew and I were trying to lend a hand to our siblings, we had few people to share our anxieties with; we didn't even have much to read that wasn't either a fringe article or a medicalized profile. And there were too many times we saw mistreatment and a lack of resources.

A World Psychiatric Association study launched in Alberta in 1996 found that the most effective way to change attitudes and remove stigma is to establish contact between people with mental health issues and other members of the public. We are grateful to the contributors who write about their families, and especially to those who share stories of personal battles, who by so doing begin to make connections. Sometimes it's said that these people are brave to share their stories, and while this may be true, it shouldn't be so. A person should not have to be brave to write about who they are. And these stories, just like life, are not all negative. There are successes, there is even some humour, and, above all, we hope you will see the strange, sweet love exuding from the stories.

This is not to say all the stories are happy. There is one in this collection of twenty-nine that entails a tragic story of violence. To some, this is the juggernaut in removing the stigma. To say violent crime has no connection to mental health is not accurate. But too often when someone who suffers from a mental illness perpetrates a crime, people don't seek any further information; they think they know why it happened. It's the illness and that's the end of it. In some cases, it's the media that skews the issue. A violent crime occurs and it's reported that the perpetrator is mentally ill. Whether any psychiatrist has made a diagnosis is not even a question. If a plane crashes, would any responsible journalist report that the pilot suffered a stroke without medical verification? In other cases, there is also a substance abuse issue, and it is the substance, not the illness, that is the cause. Add to this the fact that the substance abuse usually starts as an ineffective form of self-medication, too often because the resources to diagnose or treat have been inadequate, and the sample in the Petri dish starts to grow into an unreliable specimen. And while it is true a percentage of people with mental health issues can become violent, so can a percentage of so-called normal people. We all know certain subgroups of motorcyclists have connections to crime. To say that your friend or relative is a motorcyclist tells the world nothing about his or her propensity toward crime. It is no different for people with mental health issues.

Though we were convinced the anthology was a good thing, we had to struggle through other aspects. The closer we got to publication, the more we worried about things that for a writer should be simple, such as what to title the book. How to take the palpable stories of so many others, bundle them together, and give them a label that fits all. We had originally subtitled the book Lucid Writing on Madness. It suited us, and for a time we convinced ourselves that surely people would understand the literary reference. But eventually we came to see that many would not, and for those we would be feeding back into the stigma and fear.

Even the subtitle we settled on, True Stories from People Who Live with Mental Illness, does not sit entirely well. Although it is a plainspoken subtitle, sadly the term mental illness still carries a stigma. And although a writer such as Thomas Szasz is largely forgotten, he did have a point—to use a term such as disease or illness to describe a human condition does not see those who are living with the situation as people first. Lastly, there is much debate as to whether some of the topics addressed in this anthology—autism, post-traumatic stress disorder, and depression—are mental illnesses or something else. Indeed, if R.D. Laing was correct, even the psychosis of schizophrenia is not an illness; it is the only sane way to reconcile the horror of death that looms at the end of all our personal tunnels. Not wanting to play out the entire history of modern-day psychiatry in the quest for a title, suffice it to say that the subtitle we chose was in the end a compromise.

We hope this anthology engages you and helps you to make some connections. If you can, please consider attending a NAMIWalk or participating in a Canadian Mental Health Association event during Mental Health Week. We're all in this together.

Aftermath

FIONA TINWEI LAM

She takes herself out on walks
a few times a week,
and tells herself to finish
her vegetables.

She keeps herself away
from people who won't understand
her bond with the ceiling,
the therapeutic value of lying in bed
for a month.

If she's good,
she escorts herself out
on a day pass, feigns normalcy
over a cup of decaf.

It's so much like a golf course,
manicured and green
with roses on the fringe
of the parking lot
so no one notices

the barbed wire artfully
braided into the hedges.

Wellspring

Bad Day

JOEL YANOFSKY

All I can think of is the old joke. The one about the man who's told he has six months to live. "I want a second opinion," he says. "Okay," his doctor replies, "you're ugly too." I laugh despite myself, an involuntary snicker, and my wife frowns at me. She knows me well enough by now to know that this is what I do, make jokes at inappropriate moments. But she also has reason to expect that, under the circumstances, I'd give it a rest. We are waiting, my wife and I, for a second opinion—or a child psychiatrist to confirm the diagnosis of a previous psychologist, the one who informed us that our four-year-old son, Jonah, has autism.

My wife ignores my joke and returns to her magazine, *Exceptional Family*. "Listen," she eventually says and reads me a passage from the magazine's editorial about "blessings in disguise." Now, it's my turn to suppress the urge to roll my eyes. There are days we hardly recognize each other, my wife and I. We have become the sort of couple who indulge regularly in disapproving looks and eye-rolling. We are a new kind of family. We are exceptional.

Quite the euphemism, I almost say, but I restrain myself. You won't read this in any magazine, but when you are the parent of an "exceptional child" this is the first lesson you learn: never ever say what you are thinking.

Dr. G is a soft-spoken woman, probably in her mid-fifties, who manages to balance kindness with detachment. It's a characteristic of the mental health care profession I can't get used to. There are probably sound reasons for this approach, this impersonal compassion, but the only one I can think of is that it's because they know no matter what they say they are only guessing; that when it comes to figuring out human behaviour, the odds will always be stacked against them.

I also get the feeling that Dr. G wants to get this, her last appointment of the morning, over with. In any case, she has nothing new to tell us, which is what we suspected and feared just the same. She spends a few minutes examining Jonah, asking him his name, which he gets right, and asking him to identify the colour blue, which he doesn't. Mostly though, there's a long list of questions for us.

Does he rock back and forth?

No.

Does he flap his hands?

No.

Have we had his hearing tested? Yes. Have we been to a speech pathologist? Yes again.

We pass, or more likely fail, this test as Jonah jumps happily on a small trampoline in the corner of the office. "Mommy, Mommy," he shouts, "give me a bad day."

Jonah's speech is fine; it just doesn't always make sense to other people. When he asks for a bad day, for instance, he's really asking for a story *about* a bad day. Typically, he wants one he's heard before, a story that will have lots of characters falling down and feeling sad. He greets the accumulation of bad news by pretending to cry, but his glum expression hides an adorably unsympathetic smile. He has always been quirky and we have always loved his quirkiness. Now, we will have to learn to call it something else.

Pervasive developmental disorder, or PDD, was the label the first psychologist used. That's revised this morning to the more encompassing autism spectrum disorder, or ASD, most likely high-functioning, though Dr. G does not mention what that means in specifics. Instead she focuses on what we have to be grateful for. He talks. He makes eye contact. He is affectionate. He seems happy and good-natured. With luck and hard work, he will go to school, though he may always need support. The recommended treatment for autism is applied behavioural analysis, or ABA, but we might also want to look into relationship development intervention, or RDI. There are also books we can buy, diets we can consider—more experts we can talk to.

"I know it's a lot to absorb," Dr. G says. "The learning curve can be steep."

My wife takes notes and asks a few questions. The truth is she has already done her research. She's already hired an ABA consultant and set up an intensive therapy program for our son, thirty-six hours a week. Before we leave her office, Dr. G reaches into her drawer and pulls out a photocopy of an article titled "A Trip to Holland," written by Emily Perl, the mother of a child with a developmental disability. Dr. G hands it to my wife, who glances at the article and then quickly tucks it into her copy of *Exceptional Family*.

■　■　■

My son asks again for "a bad day" on the drive home and beams when my wife indulges him. She tells him the story of Ellie the Elephant who wakes up on the wrong side of the bed in the morning, puts on the wrong trousers, and is generally disappointed every hour on the hour. Jonah listens intently, mainly so he can correct any detail my wife gets wrong, any word she might omit.

"Give me an instead of," Jonah says. By this he means include the words "instead of" in the story. For instance, Ellie ordered blueberry pancakes with syrup but "instead of" getting syrup she got mustard. There's a lesson here too: my son understands what some of us never manage to. What some of us keep forgetting. Not getting what you want is bad, yes, but it's nowhere near as bad as expecting more than you get. You want to tell a truly sad story, a crushing one, that's the component you're looking for.

In his own way, Jonah is a perfectionist, but he's a perfectionist forced to operate in a second language, one he barely understands. As a consequence, he is unnerved by change. He resists challenges. He thrives, instead, on knowing only what he knows.

In this respect, he is like all of us, only more so. When he was two he memorized the names of the fifty-two breeds of horses from a novelty deck of cards. He pronounced words like *Appaloosa* and *Lipizzaner* with ease. What we presumed, then, to be precociousness was instead an obsession with routine and repetition. He is not yet capable of a real conversation, and from everything I'm learning about autism, he may never be.

Here's something else I've learned since my son was diagnosed: he deals with disappointment the same way I do—grudgingly. Our job is to keep him from doing what he most wants to do: stay isolated in his own world. The outside world only exists for him when we, his mother and I, his team of therapists, are present to call attention to it. So, someone is always present. Someone is always pointing to a game or toy or ball, saying, "Look, Jonah." To simply engage him requires tremendous effort. He is, when it comes to the world and what it has to offer, singularly unimpressed. These days and, in this respect, he and I are more alike than different.

"So can I see it?" I ask my wife.

"See what?" We are now home and she is busy giving Jonah lunch.

"The article, the one the doctor gave us before we left."

"It's nothing, really, just something they give to everyone, I'm guessing, when—"

"When what?" I ask.

"I don't know . . . When they don't know what else to say," she says and hands me the article.

Emily Perl's "A Trip to Holland" is intended as a pep talk for parents going through the same thing the author went through. Perl acknowledges that, of course, it is a shock when you learn your child has a problem. A shock and a disappointment, too, because none of this is what you expected or planned for.

But compare your situation, she writes, to planning a trip to Italy. You learn the language, you imagine yourself visiting the Sistine Chapel or throwing coins into the Trevi Fountain. But then you learn that you have not landed in Italy but Holland instead. Nothing is the way you expected. There will be adjustments on your part, major ones. But—

"But what?" I ask my wife. I stop reading. Instead, I am contemplating throwing something, a plate or a vase seems about right, but I am a civilized man, if not an especially mature one, so I pick up an orange and throw it at the kitchen wall.

"But we're not in fucking Holland," I say, and my wife glares at me. I forgot that Jonah is in the room. My wife pats him on the head and drags me into the bathroom, closing the door behind her and folding her arms across her chest. This is an argument I will lose, I'm just not ready to lose it yet.

"Holland! Holland would be fine. Fabulous," I say, trying to keep my voice down. "Holland has tulips . . . wooden shoes . . . windmills . . . hashish . . . hookers in the window. This is not Holland. This is like thinking you were supposed to be going to Italy and you find out you're in . . . in . . . hell."

"She is just saying you have to try to, I don't know, make the best of a bad situation, that's all. You know, if life hands you lemons you—"

"You make a sourpuss," I say.

"Great."

"What do you want from me?" I ask.

"I want to know all this bitterness, all this self-pity is going to stop sometime," my wife says. "Because it doesn't help me and it doesn't help the situation. This isn't just about you. It's about our family, about our baby," my wife says, and she is close to tears, which I know I can prevent if I make a gesture, if I apologize, or put my arm around her, or just shut up.

But I do none of these things. Instead I fold *my* arms tightly across my chest, rock back and forth, and mutter. That's because, if you ask me, at this moment, it *is* all about me; all about what is being done to me, about the catastrophe, the curse I feel has descended upon my family.

One more thing I've learned since my son's diagnosis—you can break an orange. You can do this by throwing it against the wall. It will not bounce like an apple or splatter like a tomato, but a small fissure will appear in the peel and the inside will be damaged, almost imperceptibly.

■ ■ ■

The future is what you are given when you have your first child. When you are a new parent you always have a sense of something coming—a sense so perpetual, so ordinary, you can't imagine you never felt it before. Except you never did. How could you?

So you feel it and you do what people have always done: you choose names and wallpaper, you worry about disposable diapers and daycare, you buy life insurance, you daydream fifteen or twenty years down the line about colleges and girlfriends.

When you learn your child has autism, it's the future that is taken away.

■ ■ ■

There was a story in the newspaper the other day about an asteroid heading our way, one big enough to level the whole planet, which is to say the entire human race. Real-life sci-fi. Our own doomsday scenario. Finally, we can be as certain of the future as those religious fanatics who keep predicting the world will end, then have to rethink. *Did we say April 12? We meant September 4.* In this case, scientists were committing to a specific date—February 19, 2019.

I am having trouble getting that asteroid out of my thoughts. I do a Google search daily just to make sure that the big ball of gas is still on course. This is something else I can't say out loud: I want it to come. I am like a trash-talking ballplayer. *Bring it on*, I think to myself.

The ultimate bad day.

Perhaps I'm not the only one entertaining such dark thoughts. Think about it: isn't this just the kind of break the whole human race is waiting for? I mean, really, what a way to go, everyone together. No one singled out for special treatment; no one left behind to grieve or feel sorry for themselves or be envious of the good fortunes of others. All of us destined to be extra-planetary fodder. A kind of socialism of mass destruction. So, *fine by me*, I think. If you're telling me that I don't have to be around to compare my heartbreak to the next guy's—well, what's not to like?

But at dinner my wife passes on a report she heard on the radio—the asteroid isn't coming after all. It has veered off course; the scientists, the experts, are admitting they're wrong. I pretend to shrug the news off. I laugh it off too, with an exaggerated swipe of my brow. *Phew*. I won't say what I am thinking, but I'm still thinking it: *Just my luck*. I feel as let down as one of those religious nuts.

"Plan B, huh?" my wife says, and I realize that for the first time in a while we're on the same wavelength. The comfort of a huge asteroid destroying the planet has been denied us. Instead, we can't kid ourselves anymore. We've already received our blow and now all that remains to be seen is if we will absorb it. And—what's even harder to predict—how we will.

■　■　■

Before bed tonight, Jonah follows his usual routine. He lines up his bedtime books so they stretch from one end of his room to the other. It's a task he takes on with the deliberateness of a chess master. He weighs each move carefully, then won't take his hand off the book he is placing in the line until it's exactly where he wants it.

Tonight, I deliberately intrude on his routine. Tonight, I pick up a copy of *Green Eggs and Ham*, the book at the end of the line, the one touching the far wall. He's not happy about this. He tries to close the book in my hand, but I hold him tightly in my lap while I read. I can feel myself gritting my teeth; I am squeezing him so tightly, so desperately.

Dr. Seuss's story is about stubbornness, of course, but it's also about persistence, so I persist. I make a pest of myself. By the time I finish the story, he is crying. But when I give him back the book to put in its proper place, he hesitates. In his expression, I can see how hard this is for him, how brave he is to make this simple gesture. I can also see how hard things will always be, how brave he will always have to be. And then he gives the book back to me and says, "Again, Daddy." *Again*, I think, indeed, again.

My wife has been listening at the door and she comes in to put her arms around me. "Sam I am," she whispers in my ear, adding, "I will hug you in the rain. And on a train. In a box. With a fox." She is joking around and I like seeing her laugh. As tempting—and as easy—as it would be to give up on the world, it is proving a lot harder to give up on this family.

"Give me a bad day," I say to her, sort of smiling myself.

"Too late for that now," she says. "Maybe tomorrow."

The Path to Sanity

JAMIE JOHNSON

The sound of a small dog's continuous bark grated on my nerves as I watched my seventeen-year-old son pace.

"You HAVE to get me out of here, Mom! I can't stay here! If I stay, something terrible will happen!"

I put my hand to my forehead and leaned into it. *If only that stupid mutt would shut up, maybe I could think.* As I tried to figure out a way to calm my son, the annoying little dog came into sight. It was a skinny, excited-looking boy in his late teens, obviously stimulated by my son's panic, and barking madly like a Pomeranian or Poodle would at strangers. *How in the world had we ended up here?*

■　■　■

For months, my son had been seeing a psychiatrist for depression. Weekly visits for therapy were part of his treatment. It had begun earlier that summer, when he was home alone and found our seventeen-year-old family pet on the floor lying in a pool of urine and vomit. She looked like a dog consumed by an evil spirit, eyes zipping back and forth uncontrollably. She was obviously dying. That must have been the kicker in an already stressful year.

The depression therapy didn't seem to be working, however. He was sleeping too much, distant, and easily irritated. Then, months into his treatment, one Friday night, as we drove through town in our car, my son looked at me shyly and said, "You keep calling me Joey. People have been doing that all day. I take it he is your son? I don't know who this Joey is, but my name's *not* Joey."

My heart stopped. The space around me closed in.

This stranger was like a passive, friendly child. He was completely innocent. Food was an exciting new experience. The town we lived in was "beautiful." His enthusiasm was so unlike my withdrawn, depressed teen. *What the hell was going on?*

Luckily, the next day, he came down the stairs as my son. *Thank you, God.* I felt like I had seen my child in a horrendous car accident that had left him skewered with a metal rod. He was alive and safe. He was okay . . . but would he stay that way? He definitely had some sort of gaping hole that needed mending.

Monday rolled around without any more strangeness. We drove toward Joey's weekly appointment in the city, listening to music on the way. Normally, I would be singing along, but that day I was quiet. I wondered what his doctor's reaction would be to our Friday night story. I privately prayed that it wouldn't create the need to start over with a new doctor.

Halfway there, I felt a pair of eyes. I looked over to see Joey watching me, a strangely affectionate expression on his face. He smiled.

I smiled back.

I turned from him to the road. He was still watching me, I could feel it. I looked over at him again, waiting for him to say what he was thinking. He looked at peace, like a kid again, as if we'd just spent the day together—playing foosball, going to a movie, finishing with a game of mini-putt. At that moment, all the tension of the summer was gone.

With obvious affection, he said, "I've missed you."

That threw me even more. I stumbled, "What? What do you mean?"

Still wearing that innocent, satisfied expression, he said, "It feels like it's been a long time."

Apparently, his mind was on holidays again.

Smiling gently, he said, "How are Cuddles and Licky?"

He was referring to our cats, one of which had died years before. I hesitated a second and said, "Joe . . . Licky's gone."

A gloomy look washed over his face. "Oh," he said and sat silent for a second. Then he added, "I miss them too." His head tilted down in sadness. His expression changed to fear almost immediately.

We are certainly going to have more than the Friday night story to talk to Dr. M about.

Filled with dread, I repeatedly glanced from the road to Joey. He looked totally freaked out. With eyes as wide as two full moons, he held his hands out in front of himself and asked, "Why are my hands so big?"

"Because you're seventeen, honey."

His confused reply was simply, "I am? How?"

It was the strangest thing. Although he looked the same as always, at the same time, he didn't. His features had taken on an innocence. The look on his face was so sweet.

But his voice was filled with panic. "Oh . . . my body is big too! What's happening, Mommy? What's going on?"

He hadn't called me Mommy in years.

"I'm not sure, honey, but we're on our way to see a doctor. He'll know and he will explain. Don't worry, everything will be all right."

At seventeen, Joey was a typical teenager who knew *everything* and acted like his parents knew nothing. This boy in front of me was nowhere close to seventeen and openly needed my help. His eyes pleaded for answers. I had to fight to keep my composure. I was used to Joey keeping his feelings safely protected from sight. This new, fragile appearance made my heart pain. He sat staring at his hands, obviously dumbstruck at the appearance of himself. Then he looked over at me and eked out, "Mommy, I'm really scared."

I cooed reassurances. "It's okay, honey. It's all right. Everything's going to be fine." Inside I was thinking that it was the strangest thing I had ever seen or heard. From just his voice and his language, I would have guessed him to be somewhere around seven or eight years old. When I was able to force my eyes back to the road, it was like I was listening to an old recording of him.

But as shaken as I felt, he appeared even worse. I took the steering wheel with my left hand, offered him my right, and said, "Do you want to hold my hand until we get there?" I was amazed by my automatic response. It didn't make sense for me to ask my seventeen-year-old if he wanted to hold my hand. It was just that he really didn't seem that old.

He smiled sweetly and put his hand in mine. I hoped that holding my hand was helping him because it was making me feel totally rattled. I had offered my hand to calm him, but it had done the opposite for me. I took deep breaths, trying to remain calm. *You're almost there, Jamie. Hold it together. Concentrate on the traffic.*

Although reeling with apprehension, another less intense feeling was there as well. I couldn't help but think about how nice the warmth of his hand felt, as if I were experiencing a memory I could actually feel. But mixed with this feeling of longing for a simpler day was dread. *Why was this happening? What would cause his brain to suddenly jump back ten years?*

I was in heavier traffic now, making my way through the city toward the psychiatric hospital and Dr. M. Joey suddenly looked very curious. His eyes widened as he said, "Mommy, can I see my face?"

I wondered what the sight of his face would do to him. The look of his hands had made him so nervous. His face might send him into a panic attack. Struggling to keep my voice natural, I said, "We're almost there, honey. There are mirrors in the washrooms where we're going."

Although a bit disappointed with my answer, he seemed to settle a little.

I squeezed my car into one of the few empty spots at the hospital and kept a close watch as we crossed the pavement toward the big brick building. His movements were childlike, more peppy and animated than that of a teenager.

We entered Dr. M's waiting area. At one side were the restrooms. The sight of the stick man on the men's room door brought excitement to Joey's face. "Can I go to the bathroom, Mommy?"

"Okay," I said, "but come right back." I was surprised at how I couldn't help but answer him as if he were young again. It was all too weird. As I sat down in one of the stiff waiting room chairs, I desperately prayed that the doctor was on schedule.

Joey came out of the restroom without his glasses. He needed his glasses to be able to see across the room. They were the first thing he reached for when he got up in the morning. Today he walked toward me without them.

I held back more amazed apprehension and said, "Joey, where are your glasses?"

He didn't answer. He simply patted his pocket to tell me they were safe inside.

I was totally mesmerized. Before his teen years, Joey had continually taken his glasses off and put them in his pocket. Keeping them on his face had been a constant battle. He had broken so many pairs that way, I had lost count. Somehow, my son was a young boy again. How in the world would we deal with this if it happened again? *What if it happened at school?*

■ ■ ■

Dr. M looked up from his papers as we entered his tiny office, his face curious at my presence in the room. I explained that we had a situation that needed a little clarification, and I was going to try to help. We sat down as I recounted the events of Friday night and then described what had taken place in the car. I struggled in the end, saying finally, "His personality seems to be . . . fragmenting."

Dr. M looked at Joey intently and began to ask questions.

Out of the corner of my eye, I saw Joey go limp. Both of us

watched as his body slumped, his arms dangled at his sides, his head bent forward, chin to chest, as if totally and deeply asleep yet sitting up.

After about half a minute, he looked up and blinked nervously, aware that he was being stared at by both of us. He looked from me to Dr. M, and back to me, with questions behind his eyes.

Dr. M asked if he remembered what had happened.

As Joey answered, I knew my teenaged son was back. The last thing he could recall was being in the car and driving toward the city. He had lost forty-five minutes completely.

The discussion that followed was one of options.

Dr. M looked at Joey. "Do you think you are okay to go home?" he asked.

Joey replied, "I don't know. I guess so." His eyes shifted nervously between me and Dr. M.

I turned to look at Joey. I was about to ask if that was what he wanted. Before I could get the question out, his body went limp again. His head fell down to his chest, and his arms went lifeless.

I looked at Dr M. I'd hoped he would offer some insight, or words of comfort. Instead he looked back at me with lifted eyebrows, appearing as confused as I was.

Slowly, Joey lifted his head. His facial expression was different again. This time, he had an air of total confidence. His features crinkled into a creepy little smile. In a strange, arrogant manner, he said, "What's going on?" and tilted his head slightly to one side as if amused.

Dr. M answered with, "We are trying to decide if you need to go into the hospital or not."

With an intimidating stare, Joey slowly exhaled. "Hmm . . . I see."

He looked at me, his eyebrows lowered, his eyes intense and glaring.

I was scared. It might sound strange, but this person beside me did not feel one bit like Joey. I had gone from worried and confused to completely rattled, to now panicked, all within an hour, without one minute of relief in between.

Dr. M's eyes remained fixed on Joey. He announced he needed a second opinion. There was a doctor on the hospital staff he thought might have some insight. He dialled the phone and sat waiting as it rang, watching Joey carefully.

Joey looked at him and smiled his wry little grin again. Then he turned his attention back to me. He leaned in and whispered, "Get out of here, Jamie," his eyes piercing me.

My blood pressure shot through the roof. His intimidating, forceful stare actually made me want to get out of there. I didn't think I could handle much more.

Dr. M was talking on the phone now, asking questions. I heard him say, "I was wondering if he should go into the hospital until he has better control."

Joey looked away from me for a minute and with an amused smile said, "Oh, don't worry. It's me that is in total control here." He gave a low, grating snicker that sent a shiver right through me.

He looked back at me again, his head tilted down so that his offensive stare looked even more intimidating. He said confidently, "Run, Jamie, run. Get out of here. If someone gets hurt, I don't want it to be you." His calmness was frightening.

My eyes shifted to Dr. M. The tears I had been fighting became too massive to hold back. A wet trail quickly lined each of my cheeks. I couldn't think. What had happened to my Joey? I looked back at him, unable to believe this was happening, but quickly turned away. Looking at him sent fear through my system. It was too much to bear. I couldn't look at this sinister person. A small sob slipped out.

Joey's voice got a little louder this time "Run, Jamie. Run." Anger trembled in his voice.

The next voice I heard was Dr. M's. "Never mind. Send someone over to take him . . . I'm putting him in."

■ ■ ■

I sat alone in my car feeling like the supporting actress in some strange psychological thriller, desperately trying to hold myself together. I had been told to go home and return with overnight things while a guard took my son. *What had happened to him?* He wasn't violent; he had a gentle, animal-loving personality. He wouldn't even kill a bug, let alone hurt a person.

Somehow, I managed to drive home and absently pack a bag. When I returned, Joey was back, and he was *not* happy. "I can't stay here, Mom. If I stay in this place, I will really go crazy!"

But, under doctor's orders, he had to stay—he needed further evaluation. I was to come back the next day and bring more of his things to a place called Algonquin Cottage, enough things for "a while."

The look of the "cottage" did not help to rid me of the feeling I was trapped in a movie of the week. Algonquin Cottage was a perfectly round house. (Well, according to Joey, it was actually octagonal, but my memory seems to have smoothed out the edges.) It and two identical others lined the back of the property, hidden from sight all the months I had been coming to the hospital. They were the strangest-looking buildings I'd ever seen.

I knocked on the cold steel of the door, bracing myself, waiting to learn what to expect from his stay. A tall, skinny teen answered the door, followed closely by a stocky woman of fifty or so—the head nurse. Once inside, I unfortunately asked her one too many questions. "How long is the average stay for a teen like Joey?"

"Six to eight weeks."

My mouth went dry. *What?* I had been expecting one or two . . . *six to eight weeks. Oh my God.* My throat was closing. The tears were headed out fast. I stumbled out of the office and plunked down in a chair. Joey was pacing back and forth, wringing his hands. My mouth hung open. *Six to eight weeks?*

That's when the stupid little dog began barking. It was the skinny teen who had answered the door. *Jesus!*

Then I heard Joey. Terror had completely taken over his voice. In a loud, panicked plea, he roared, "Mom, do something! I *have* to get out of here. I can't be held responsible for what happens if you leave me here. I CAN'T STAY! This place will kill me!"

I looked up as he stood over me, his face scarlet with passion. I choked out, "Honey, there is nothing I can do. You can talk to the doctor tomorrow."

He yelled back, "Tomorrow? Tomorrow? I will be totally insane by tomorrow." He was in hysterics. Loud and forceful, he shouted, "If you leave me here with these crazy people, something terrible will happen. I might hurt someone. I can't stay here. Mom, you can't leave me here. If I do hurt someone, do you want *that* on your conscience?"

I bent forward in my chair. My head fell into my hands. Nothing would come out of my mouth. I rocked back and forth in my chair slightly as he shouted, not knowing what on earth to do. I had reached my limit.

Then I felt a hand rest softly on my shoulder. I looked up to see the nurse. She gently said, "Jamie, this is too much. You don't have to hear this. It's time for you to go home." She took her hand off my shoulder and gently lifted me out of the chair.

There was another caregiver between Joey and me by then, a young man, preventing Joey from stopping me. I let the nurse guide me to the exit. I felt completely numb, like I had been drugged.

Joey broke free from the guy blocking him and ran toward me. The young caregiver dashed after him but heard his superior say, "Let him go."

My son threw his arms around me and sobbed into my shoulder. He clung to me as if he would never see me again. Through his sobs, I heard him say, "Oh Mom, I am so, so sorry . . . I'm so sorry . . . I'm so sorry."

I couldn't speak. We just stood there holding each other, crying.

We stayed that way for several minutes, letting the pain fade. Then I heard in a soft voice, "I'm so sorry, Mom. I didn't mean it. I love you."

My voice thickened with emotion as I murmured, "It's okay, honey . . . I know. I love you too."

■　■　■

My son spent that year with five extra personalities. He was under hospital care for the first two months and was diagnosed with disso-ciative identity disorder (DID). Doctors say the condition is usually caused by repetitive childhood abuse and only resurfaces when that child is older and suffers too much stress.

It was awful to think that Joey may have suffered something horrifying. For months my thoughts ran terrible scenes through my mind. What type of abuse? Had it been at school, while he was with a babysitter, at the playground? God, I wished my brain had an off button.

His doctors searched for this buried trauma. The key to his full recovery, without risk of his alternate personalities popping up again, was to find it and deal with it. I wanted to help, and I vowed to do whatever was necessary to find the solution.

I would walk away from his hospital room even though I desper-ately wanted to bring him home, to get him away from the stress of the other patients' attempted suicides and assorted mental illnesses. I would drive him to appointment after appointment and give our family history to doctor after doctor. I would put aside my fear of what the ominous "hidden memories" were in order to find them and work past them. I would deal with the skeptics, the ignorant people who thought his illness was imaginary, that his "alters" were simply a plea for attention.

My son knew his extra personalities were what kept him in the hospital, but they stuck around for his full eight-week stay . . . and for months after. He detested those weeks in the hospital, yet every once in a while, on visiting day, I'd visit with a stranger. Why would he continue his "act" when he wanted desperately to go home? The answer is simple—he didn't have a choice.

And neither did I. I needed my son to be whole again. I wouldn't give up.

That is . . . unless I was forced to.

After a year of therapy, Joey's DID specialist cut him loose. She hadn't found the memories of hidden abuse that caused his alters, but she felt Joey had better control over the other personalities and that he would be able to manage.

I felt deserted. I wanted to look for a new psychiatrist. Joey didn't. He was sick of prying appointments and it wasn't up to me. Joey was eighteen, and it was his life.

I had to learn the unthinkable: that if I've done all I can, if I've offered my knowledge, my time, my heart, and my help and nothing works, I must accept the fact that some things aren't fixable . . . and love my son for who he is, exactly the way he is.

The Last Call

JILL SADOWSKY

Friday, January 18, 1996

I brewed my morning coffee, poured some into my favourite blue mug, and sat down to scan the morning headlines in the Hebrew newspaper. The telephone rang at 8:05 AM. I leapt to answer. It was Inspector Cohen from the Petach Tikvah police station.

■ ■ ■

Our son, Doron, died three months short of his thirty-fourth birthday. This haunted being found his way to a deserted construction site and, on the coldest, wettest night of the year, threw himself off the scaffolding of an unfinished building. In reality, Doron was long gone, dying bit by bit over the sixteen-year period of his battle against paranoid schizophrenia.

For me, the question: "How many children do you have?" is a hard one to answer. Now I normally respond, "Two daughters." But I did have a son—Doron, whose life was measured by before, when he lived in the world with us, and after, the long years he lived in hell with demons tormenting him until he removed himself from both worlds, leaving a place in my heart where tears flow.

I did not understand what went wrong, when it started to go wrong. "Classic," the psychiatrists said. What did we know of this illness, classic or not? We had barely come across the name schizophrenia. In Israel, where Doron grew up, mental illness was what the shell-shocked of Holocaust survivors had to deal with, or soldiers in arms suffered from. It conjured up no images that we could remotely associate with our good-looking, strapping, six-foot first-born on his surfboard.

In a strange way, with no preconceptions and having faith in modern medicine, we understood that, like appendicitis, with the proper treatment, our son would get better. It was a medical condition, and in the same way that many cancers are resistant to some treatments and responsive to others, we were sure that Doron could be treated successfully. And mostly we understood that just as we could not cause AIDS or cancer, we could not cause schizophrenia. We put our faith in an army of psychiatrists, psychologists, social workers, occupational therapists, and orderlies.

Doron joined the Israeli army with a medical profile of 97, the highest score possible. His first cry for help came during his three-year compulsory army service when he took an overdose of pills. He'd refused to sign on to do an officer's course and was coerced into doing so. Incredibly, he was returned to his unit despite his misery. Oh, if we had only known how miserable he'd been. He received his honourable discharge at the age of twenty-one from his unit on schedule, with a reduced profile of course.

He started and stopped various business ventures, which didn't seem too unusual. The transition to civilian life often takes time. When he began studying at the Tel Aviv University and requested earplugs, we were impressed that he was so intent on blocking out his neighbour's radio to concentrate on his studies. How could we have known that he was trying to still the voices within his head?

I only know that after he had been hospitalized for a year, we finally heard the diagnosis. Then he was discharged. This all came as a shock; we'd had little explanation of what we were up against. We believed that Doron would emerge healthy.

He was given Thorazine, Haldol, Mellaril. He tried psychotherapy, occupational therapy, and group therapy, yet he continued to be out of focus, angry, hostile, then suddenly apathetic and listless. He stopped worrying about how he looked until he finally appeared on the outside like the wild man clawing at him from within.

Our two young daughters started shying away from their older brother. They stopped bringing friends home, visited him in the hospital less, and steered away from him at home as they suddenly became afraid of him. We started family therapy at the hospital.

"What can we do to help Doron?" we asked.

"What do you think you should do?"

"We don't know what to do when he gets violent and abusive."

"Tell us what you do."

"The girls are afraid to have friends over as we never know when Doron will start ranting or how he will react."

"*Act normally.*"

Is this what the medical professionals spent ten years in graduate school to learn?

Doron took clozapine and Risperdal, but they were not the miracle drugs we were after. We tried living with him at home, allowing him to "get on with his life," as one psychiatrist put it. Then we rented an apartment for him as no group home would take someone who was not working at least a few hours a day. We ended up paying for two homes, two cleaning persons, and two telephone lines. I was left doing our laundry at home as well as at my son's. I cooked Doron's favourite foods at home to stock his otherwise empty refrigerator and often stood by and watched as he threw out the food, convinced I was poisoning him. Sometimes he stayed in his apartment for days, filling us with dread, wondering what he was up to. Other times, he came home to crash in his old room where we worried he might suddenly turn hostile.

Meanwhile, our daughters did without: without enough time

and energy from us, without vacations or parties at home, without frills and extras where every available shekel was poured into another prescription, another treatment, a different psychiatrist. My husband and I did without too. We minded less.

We tried private, out-of-hospital doctors. We turned to friends and family for support, but it appeared that although we knew Doron was ill, to most of the world he was crazy, undeserving of much attention. Our thirteen-year-old daughter summed it up: "If Doron's body were hurting, people would send gifts, but because it is his mind, they throw bricks." Friends called less and visited less; not because they no longer cared, but because they did not know what to say. Other times, people would ask about Doron, but it always seemed to be at a time when I was desperately trying to think of something other than the ravages of his schizophrenia. How were they to know? I promised myself that one day I would write a book explaining what the appropriate things are to say to someone with a chronically ill child.

Then we were thrust into the stigma blame loop. "She's the one with the crazy son. Maybe he's crazy because she is?" I wanted to shout, "But I have healthy daughters. Are they healthy because I am?" And all the time in the background and often in the foreground, Doron was alternately withdrawn or aggressive, often tearing us apart with his recurring taunt, "I'll dance on your graves."

For sixteen years we searched for a way to help him and for sixteen years we looked for just one health care worker who would sit with us, explain things to us, guide us, and include us. I needed someone to show me that they cared. We were kept at arm's length: "Patient confidentiality, you know." Did those same doctors realize that the Doron who said such hurtful things about us said equally horrific things about them? We should have all been working as one.

At one session, Doron pulled out the grubby notebook he carried with him at all times, turned to a page in the middle, and asked me to read out a poem he'd written.

Autumn is drawing near
Soon I'll see the leaves falling.
Autumn, I am waiting for you
because the summer is lost.

There is no sea, no sun
no sunbathing, no swimming
Here I am, waiting for the
leaves to fall from the trees
to symbolize winter's arrival.

And so, spring, summer, autumn, winter
I'm stuck in the same place.
Doctors refuse to help me
and leave me in the same spot.

The silence in that hospital office was palpable until the psychologist said, "You only speak about Doron at these family sessions." I was unable to reply as I needed to recover from what Doron had read to us.

On another visit, a psychiatric intern asked, "Don't you have problems other than Doron?" I burst out, "Don't you understand that schizophrenia is all-consuming, all-encompassing, dictating our have-to-be-coordinated timetables so that someone is always available for Doron's needs? We visit, take numerous phone calls, every day, step in when there are crises. Do you really think that we believe that this is a good, healthy way to live? Help us help Doron and then we can talk about other problems."

Then there was the social worker who vetoed Doron's participation in a workshop, but when I asked, "What can we do when he doesn't take his medication?" she answered, "I don't know. He seems to be medication resistant. Try not to upset him."

"To do that," I replied, "we'd have to avoid scratching, walking, talking out loud, moving. We'd have to allow him to live with the stench of urine in the bathroom, sheets that are never laundered."

"Oh," she added, "and you must never let him hurt you."

"I am five-foot-six. And weigh one hundred and twenty pounds. My daughters are thirteen and sixteen. My husband's strength comes from within; besides, he's at work during the day. Perhaps you should send us a supply of pre-filled syringes and teach us how to knock him out the way an orderly does in the hospital when he gets agitated."

To this day I have no idea how we were supposed to deal with Doron at his *craziest*. After sixteen years, we realized that the only options all the trained professionals were offering had nothing to do with medical science. The first was to keep a straitjacket and two orderlies around the house. The second was to call the police.

And, oh, how many times we had to call the police. Then there were the times they called us, like when Doron suddenly threw a large boulder at a passing car or hit an elderly woman on the bus. Does anyone have an idea of what it takes for a mother to come to the conclusion that she is so powerless to deal with her child that she has to turn on him and then turn him in to preserve whatever sanity she has left to protect the rest of her family? So we called the police. And followed the forced hospitalizations, the hearings, the warrants, and the reviews, all ending in the same place: a straitjacket, two orderlies, and a hypodermic.

One day Doron yelled, "I don't take medication because I'm ill, I'm ill because I take medication." Nonetheless, he started to take it religiously, desperate to get well, unable to sleep without it, lethargic and sleepy even when awake.

In retrospect, I don't know how it was possible but the word *chronic* only crept into the diagnosis years later.

Eventually I discovered how many families are torn apart by the "identified patient." I discovered how many marriages dissolve as blame and guilt become the parents' daily fare. Our family held together, sometimes barely, but then, we never for a moment felt that we were to blame, that anybody was guilty. Too many families living with a schizophrenia sufferer are consumed with both. And, too often, the doctors seem to assume that they should feel that way even as they try to help them work it through. I wonder whether they make parents of cancer patients feel bad.

Despairing of professionals, we joined a parents' support group. We met in a bomb shelter and sat in a semicircle with other parents. Every single one of them knew what Doron's illness was doing both to him and to our family. We shared our grief, anger, feelings of helplessness and hopelessness freely with them.

A year later, it became clear how much we needed the group, but it was difficult for us to express our deepest feelings in Hebrew. So, we started a self-help support group for English speakers who were sharing our hell. We opened under the auspices of ENOSH, the Israeli Mental Health Association. Before long, our numbers swelled to twenty as the ENOSH social workers wondered what damage we might be doing behind closed doors. None of us wanted a professional to run the group, although we did consult a social worker when we felt the need. We also invited the odd psychiatrist or psychologist to talk to us, but as they had little practical advice to offer in the field of coping with a mentally ill child, we changed direction.

The session on humour was very successful as it showed us how to deflect tension. We invited someone to teach us relaxation techniques. We encouraged the healthy siblings of our sick children to talk to the group about living with a mentally ill brother or sister. We cried with them, we listened and learned. They begged us not to push them to seek help as they had sat by watching us all drag our sick child from one doctor to another with little success. They insisted that if and when they needed psychological guidance, they would ask for it.

The group helped me deal with the terrible anger I was carrying around inside that was destroying me. I was angry at Doron, at the doctors, and at all the people who did not understand our grief and who so often said the wrong thing.

The director of Doron's hospital asked us to talk to his staff. Our main message: work with the parents, help them fight the stigma accorded mental illness. Teach them to take one day at a time. Make sure that every parent knows they did not cause schizophrenia no matter what society and some professionals may imply. Recognize the regret that parents have when they realize they never got a real chance to say goodbye to their child—Doron had disappeared into his illness so imperceptibly.

I hope health care workers learn the importance of a kind word and the need to offer hope to the patient and family in continual crisis. No one can live without hope. If the general readership gains insight and compassion for the plight of a family coping with mental illness, Doron's plea for us to understand his demons will not have been in vain.

■ ■ ■

Three times, Doron, which means *a gift*, tried to take his life. Three times he stockpiled the pills doled out under *close supervision* in the hospital. My Doron, my beautiful son whom I'd carried in my womb for nine months, to whom I gave life and what I thought was the promise of a good life, tried to kill himself over and over. He wanted to get better. He wanted a girlfriend, someone to love who would love him. But most of all, he needed peace of mind.

Three months short of his thirty-fourth birthday, my son finally came to the conclusion that the Doron who had been sparring with demons for sixteen years would never know that peace of mind again. So he threw himself to what we can only hope is a place of calm, peace, and endless waves fit for a surfer.

We love you, Doron, rest.
1962–1996

Stormtrooper

DELL CATHERALL

"Damn it. I deserve something."

It's been three weeks since my son's release from Vancouver General Hospital and I can still hardly understand his words. Delivered in the thinnest of monotones, they're a weak response to my warning, "These guys aren't going to hand over anything without a fight. Who knows what gang they're with? Do you really want to challenge them in the courts?"

Dylan glowers; his eyes say what his voice can't. His jaw is wired shut. He breathes like a stormtrooper from *Star Wars* and mumbles like Hannibal Lecter. He winces when he smiles or frowns. Chewing is impossible. Even drinking through a straw is forbidden, because it strains muscles trying to heal. If Dylan wants something, he grunts and points.

"Your son's lucky, Mrs. Catherall," the ambulance attendants told us the night Dylan was admitted to Vancouver General. "There were plainclothes policemen patrolling in the vicinity and they pulled off three large attackers who were punching him senseless."

In the next breath, almost like they wanted to get all the bad stuff out at once, one asked if we were aware of our son's drug use. When my husband, Greer, and I nodded, she added, "Then you won't be surprised to know we found fresh track marks on his left arm."

But we were a bit. Dylan had been smoking crack, not shooting up. At least that's what we'd let ourselves believe. He'd been living at our home for a year, and although nothing is ever easy, there'd been relative peace until this recent crisis. Four months earlier we'd laid out the conditions for his return: find a job, bathe daily, stop using cocaine, speak the truth. In the first week, Dylan ignored all our rules. What were we thinking? Our demands were surreal for an addicted kid with a bipolar diagnosis.

Dylan picked up a construction job immediately. But he was on site for only two shifts when he twisted his ankle during an anxiety attack. Embarrassed and afraid, he never went back. Our rules about his personal hygiene would have been fine ten years ago, when he was a child; now they were meaningless. He couldn't quit cocaine because it was one of the few things that momentarily released him from depression. And lying became second nature to him—an addict's survival tactic. Greer and I eventually reached a compromise with Dylan: volunteer at Coast Mental Health facility two times a week, take a shower every three days, never smoke crack in the house. The truth—Greer and I tried to stop asking questions we knew would elicit lies.

For a while things were better. Dylan tried to sit with us for at least fifteen minutes during dinnertime. He began visiting the library every Tuesday, a place that had never let him down. There were no requests for extra money. Dylan did his own laundry and took out the garbage. But Greer and I have learned to expect the worst and knew it was inevitable our son would soon find new means of stimulation.

Dylan waited. His opportunity slipped through the mailbox two weeks later: a Visa application. It was so easy: the credit limit was under five thousand dollars, so Visa didn't check Dylan's credit and employment history or dig into his past. It was all just words on paper for Dylan. A month later, Greer and I opened the first CIBC statement bearing Dylan's name. He owed $818.32. This was not the first time he'd tried a similar scam, but it was the last we'd tolerate.

I went into robot mode and calmly packed his hockey bag. Triplets of everything: underpants, shirts, hankies (the methadone makes him sweat), socks, hoodies. And the basics: shampoo, a towel, soap, Uremal for his feet (they suffer the most when you live on the street), granola bars, gift cards for Subway and Starbucks. At least he'd be okay for a while. I congratulated myself for taking a stand. It was up to him now.

When Dylan came home I ordered him to sit at the kitchen table. I showed him the invoice, explained that we were following through this time, and pointed out the hockey bag.

"You fucking bitch!"

He left without a second glance at the survival kit I'd just packed.

I had no regrets when I heard the door slam. It wasn't my fault he chose to leave empty-handed. This was what my support group had been urging me to do for months. "Set your boundaries and be firm. Giving in to his demands is not healthy for either of you."

When Greer came home at dinnertime, I was overcome with guilt. Where would Dylan sleep? How could he function without his meds? Had I gone too far?

We didn't hear anything for five days. Greer buried himself in work and spent his spare time nurturing the plants in his greenhouse. I cleaned the house non-stop and then went to the gym, adding more weights and resistance until I was exhausted and dripping. We rarely spoke. We walked like zombies through the terrible silence. We took Ativan nightly, drank too much wine, and willed the phone to ring. When it did, Greer and I weren't prepared for the call from an admitting nurse at VGH Emergency, "We have your son and he's calling for his parents."

■ ■ ■

Within thirty minutes I was beside Dylan's stretcher. This sobbing child of mine who rarely let me touch him buried his bloody face in my arms and refused to let go. I couldn't speak or cry. I rocked him like an infant.

A young police officer asked Greer if he was Dylan's father. Greer could only nod. "We got the guys that did this," the police officer said. "They're spending the night in jail, charged with aggravated assault. The police are treating this very seriously."

I looked up. "What did Dylan do?"

The officer shook his head. "Absolutely nothing. Three very drunk East Indians from Surrey had just come out of the sports bar at Hemlock and Broadway; the Canucks were knocked out of the playoffs and these goons were looking for a fight. We have a witness, says your son was walking alone, head down, minding his own business. Does he live with you?"

I pried myself from Dylan's grip so I could shake the police officer's hand and thank him. I had become the family spokesperson after the Catheralls imploded eight years earlier, the one who best buried guilt and could present the calm, cool face of reason. I gave the police officer an abbreviated account of our son's recent slide. He was empathetic and supportive and said that he'd visit Dylan at our home to help him complete a victim statement form. His two-way radio blared, "Constable Gomez report to Granville and 12th, victim attacked at bank ATM."

As Constable Gomez passed my son's stretcher, he put his hand on Dylan's shoulder and said, "Stay in your shoes, young man, no one deserves this. You've had a close call; make it work for you."

I heard the hope in Constable Gomez's voice. It made me hope, too, for the first time in I don't know how long. Could Dylan's assault be that elusive bottom, the epiphany that would start his journey to sobriety?

I went back and cradled Dylan as Greer wiped away the blood. A man in his late thirties beside me gestured in Dylan's direction. "I've been where he is. He's lucky, you know, to have parents that care. You don't want him out on that street. Ain't like it used to be. Some addicts today would kill for a rock. And the gangs carry weapons—knives, explosives, semi-automatics. I figure those rag-tops that got your son woulda finished him off good if that cop didn't show."

I agreed that our family was very fortunate that Dylan got off so lightly—nothing really, just a broken jaw. But as my neighbour continued to tell me about his litany of close calls, arrests, and unending visits to detox and the psych ward, I knew only too well my son walked the same path. Would there be a time years from now when Dylan would lie here alone because we'd given up? Or would he be alone because we'd grown old and died and there was no one left who would care?

I whispered to Greer, "This guy says he's been clean a year, but look at his pupils and the way his hands shake. He's full of it."

"Don't be so harsh, Dell, I hear something more. For all his bravado I believe he's sincere about parents making a difference. Us being here tonight is what Dylan will remember, not the fact we put him out."

"I wish I shared your optimism."

We were surprised to be visited by a doctor who wanted to dis-cuss Dylan's methadone. She assured us he would be given his usual dose the next morning. She asked if we'd noticed any changes in his behaviour since he started taking Seroquel for his bipolar disorder. *Finally here was a doctor who was willing to talk to me.* I launched into a detailed description of Dylan's latest manic episode. But I couldn't talk for long. As the cocaine and morphine wore off, Dylan began to flail his arms and legs.

Dylan tried to yell for help through his mouthful of broken teeth. He twisted from my grasp and struggled to yank the IV from his arm. With Herculean strength, he threw Greer to the floor as hospital staff rushed to constrain him. All we could do was watch as they forced Dylan into a straitjacket. Within minutes he was tethered to the stretcher. They jabbed a hypodermic deep into his thigh. As he began to relax, I wondered how much of the original Dylan was still there, how much of him was just chemicals.

■ ■ ■

My mind drifted back to the havoc of our lives six years earlier, when I had to face a young woman staffing the information desk at Langara College. I was a mess. Too skinny, shoulders slumped, barely able to hold myself together, I wanted to yell at the euphoric young people around me to shut up so I could attend to my business and get out of there. I had just taken the bus from the psychiatric ward at VGH. The day before, after trying to end his life by slitting his wrists, Dylan had driven my Camry full speed into a Downtown Eastside dumpster. I held a letter from his psychiatrist, which stated that due to recent suicide attempts Dylan Catherall was unable to attend any classes this semester. When I passed it across the counter and told the young woman Dylan would be officially withdrawing, I hoped that any failing marks wouldn't appear on his transcript because Dylan wanted to transfer into political science at the University of British Columbia. As she recorded our family's horror in Dylan's file, the girl looked up and said, "Oh, I'm so sorry; should I take his name off all class lists?"

All I could do was shrug and will the tears to stay in my eyes.

Dylan has never gone back to school of any sort; he probably never will.

■ ■ ■

"Mr. and Mrs. Catherall, we're wheeling Dylan down to radiology. Shouldn't be too long. There's a decent coffee lounge in the Pattison Pavilion; give yourselves a break."

Over tea Greer and I tried to piece together the events that led to Dylan's recent spiral. It was only five days ago that I'd opened the CIBC invoice; Dylan had been using his card for one month and that was the time we started hearing about Tricia. The signs had been there, but we'd totally missed them.

The first night he'd met this new girl, Dylan had come home late, but excited, and uncharacteristically positive about the evening. "Mom, I know it's past my curfew, but I was having a ball, really fitting in. Do you know what it's like to have friends again?"

We were happy for him and agreed to be flexible. We accepted his story and hoped these "friends" would bolster his confidence, bring him up from the basement.

The next morning Dylan didn't come back and watch cartoons after his methadone. He always said he needed at least two hours for the effects to kick in. At noon he called. "Mom, you won't believe this. I'm at Coast and I've just given my first speech in group. It was incredible; the others actually noticed me. I won't be home for dinner, I'm stopping at Chapters and buying the new manga, and then I'm going out to eat with this girl."

I wondered where all this energy was coming from. Dylan had actually risen off the couch; he was making decisions and following through. Greer and I were lulled into believing our son was finally taking a few tentative steps out of the shadows. He called again at 10:00 PM: "Mom, guess what, I just went to this rib place Tricia knows and had all the meat I could eat. I'm going to be late, sorry. I'll cut the grass tomorrow to make it up."

He wasn't late. He never came home. The phone call in the morning was alarming. "Mom, I'm working on moving in with Tricia. She goes to university and she really likes me. Sorry, can't cut the grass, Tricia's got a car and I've got a ride downtown. I'll be gone soon, you'll be happy."

I knew perfectly well that in the real world no girl is going to invite a penniless, mentally ill cocaine addict into her bed no matter how endearing he may appear on the surface.

Dylan phoned again that day, in the late afternoon. "Mom, you've got to help. I've lost my pack, my bus pass, my keys—everything. I'm using this guy's phone; come pick me up."

My first inclination was to follow instructions and bring him home, but I knew he must at least try to work it through himself.

I spoke calmly. "Dylan, think back. When was the last time you remember opening your pack to get something? Did you have it when you left Tricia?"

"Mom, how in the hell am I supposed to know. Just friggin' get in the car. I'm freezing and hungry."

"Dylan, you know I'm not going to do that right now. Where's your friend Tricia? I think you should check with her."

"That's just like you, Mom. You never care. You're always thinking of yourself and too fucking lazy to come."

Nothing more. He'd hung up the borrowed cell.

■　■　■

As we walked back to the ER, Greer and I tried to rewrite the script. If only we'd known about the bogus credit card. Access to money had always been the first trigger to set Dylan off. I berated myself for not intercepting the Visa application from CIBC. My usually calm husband looked exasperated: "Get a grip, Dell. This isn't about you, and what you did or didn't do. It's about Dylan's screw-ups. When are you going to step back and stop being some kind of martyr?"

We ran into Dylan's plastic surgeon. He'd studied the X-rays and assured us Dylan would have jaw reconstruction the next day. There was a good chance all his teeth could be saved. We were thankful. Dylan doesn't bear the physical wounds of an addict. Although his teeth are yellow through neglect, he has them. Considered a catch in high school, there was never any shortage of girlfriends. Dylan sang solos in the choir, practised Kyokushin karate, and wrote stories that shocked his creative writing class—sensitive and dangerous; girls were attracted to that. Tricia probably felt the same.

Four days after his hospitalization, we took Dylan home. At first he was thankful for every pill I crushed and every smoothie I blended. He let me hug him daily. He didn't seem too traumatized by the beating and walked seven blocks by himself each morning to London Drugs for his methadone. He co-operated with Constable

Gomez, who helped him complete the victim impact forms. He even allowed me to accompany him to an appointment with his mental health workers.

And then the second credit card statement arrived. Greer and I were shocked at Dylan's wild spending spree and sexual adventure. He went through five thousand dollars in two weeks. A hotel on Broadway, numerous cash advances, meals, and, of course, drugs. I kept wondering how I so totally missed the arc of Dylan's mania. By the time I had packed the hockey bag and put him out, he was frightened, angry, and miserable—drowning in his own obnoxious behaviour. When Greer and I showed the second invoice to Dylan, he went berserk. It took him right back to the night of the attack.

■   ■   ■

It's been three weeks since my son's release from Vancouver General Hospital and I can hardly understand him. He hides in the basement and obsesses about his attackers. They bang inside his head, pushing at his brain with fists and feet that bring delusions and nightmares. Dylan panics about his ever-increasing CIBC debt and rails against me for refusing to pay it off. He plans to sue the thugs who jumped him and collect thousands. This troubles Greer and me. My friends working in the legal system share our concern. They claim we can't expect the law to protect Dylan and us against gang retribution. The popular advice is to stay below their radar. The three attackers are charged with aggravated assault and face a court date early in the fall. We advise Dylan to declare bankruptcy, testify at the criminal trial, and forget about pressing for personal compensation. Of course he refuses with all the singlemindedness of a stormtrooper.

Raising Julie

SARA DEMETER

1993

Julie comes and sits on my knee. She hugs me hard and covers my face with big, smacking baby kisses. "I love you, Mummy," she says. She wriggles in delight, like a child at Christmas. "Oh, Mummy, I'm going to have a jacket with my name on it, just like the big kids. It's going to be—" she pauses and, with an effort that's artful and studied and should be altogether charming, says, "b—beeyoo—ti—ful!"

Julie is twenty-two, taller and heavier than I am. She has her junior bronze medal in figure skating and two-thirds of a university degree. She's won academic scholarships and public speaking trophies and was voted her school newspaper's best copy editor. Julie herself is beautiful. Charming. Helpless. Overbearing. Manipulative. Exasperating.

Julie has schizophrenia.

A Sunday's child, a Taurus, much younger than her siblings, Julie was everyone's pet at home. Her sister and brothers brought their friends to the maternity ward to admire her through the window, took part in raising her until they left home one by one.

When Julie was a toddler, her father and I thought we were doing everything right. Surely Number Four would prove we had parenthood down to a fine art. Julie walked and talked early, was curious but exceptionally careful and meticulous. Although shy, she was a joiner, determined to try everything, to learn and excel. As she grew, it became obvious that she was acquisitive, reluctant to share, afraid of people but paradoxically could shine before an audience. In adolescence she grew increasingly competitive, resentful of others' successes, and distressed over what she perceived as her insurmountable faults. She hated her nose, her blond hair; wept over marks that were lower than A and labelled herself the school's worst athlete when she came second in a race. A typical adolescent girl, we thought, typical growing pains. But a self-starter who knew where she was going and how to get there. Totally unlike her father's sister, constantly under psychiatric care, on antipsychotics.

By the time Julie was ready for high school, our stable world had been destroyed by separation, divorce, and a move to another city. Her sister married, her brothers went off to university. Left to pick up the pieces and start over, I made a fateful mistake. I put Julie in a private school, a haven from our chaos, I thought. For three years, it appeared that I was right. Happy and popular, she won scholarships, made the honour roll.

■　■　■

Her friend Trevor phones one day while she's out. He hasn't talked to her since school, didn't *know* until now. "She was the most brilliant of us all," he says. He sounds so much older than I remember, and he's sad, there's an infinite sadness in his voice, he's put her into the context of irretrievable past. Trevor's a survivor, working on his master's, aiming for the diplomatic service. She's a casualty, he says, of a private school system that was harsh and puritanical, forgiving on minor infractions but invoking the wrath of God on mortal sins: dyed hair, rock music, boy-girl relationships. In her last year at the school, Julie broke all the rules: dyed her hair black, played rap tapes, dated.

We could blame the school. Or divorce, dislocation, single-parent family. We could blame genetics. But what's the point? Blame is another chapter—not part of survival. Julie won't talk about the school. "She says she doesn't remember," Trevor says. What matters, what we have to focus on, is not the blame, but on how Julie will cope with the rest of her life. "She tells me nothing, Trevor," I say. She never did.

▪ ▪ ▪

Just before midnight on August 18, 1993, my son called from Julie's bachelor apartment in Montreal. "You'd better come," Donnie said. "Julie needs you." He lived a few blocks from her. It was 3:00 AM when I arrived, after a search for an all-night gas station and a two-hour drive. She was sleeping. "I gave her a sedative," Donnie said. "She hasn't eaten or slept for days. She told me she walks all night, and she never needs food." He shook his head. "She just got accepted into film studies at Concordia for September." We packed her bags and in the morning I drove her home to Ottawa.

Having worked in a psychiatric hospital facility, I was wary of the patient care system. Brusque, impersonal, regimented, sometimes punitive. Hit-and-miss drug treatments. Indifferent follow-up. Revolving-door policy. And wasn't it for the chronically, hopelessly mentally ill? This was my Julie!

I planned to keep her at home. Over the next three days, I bought vitamins and health foods, rubbed her back and feet, talked and read to her, cradled her in my arms. But she couldn't sleep, couldn't keep still. Astrology had taken over her life, enthralling, terrifying, overwhelming her. People were making signs that the end of the world was near. The moon was following her. "Help me," she begged. "I don't know where I leave off and the world begins."

On the fourth day, at 4:00 AM, she ran outside, barefoot in driving rain, screaming that she was going to commit suicide because her friend Sunshine was getting an Academy Award. "I should have won," she shrieked. "It's mine! I'll kill myself!" She tore down the street in drenched pyjamas. I got the car out and drove her to the Royal Ottawa Hospital. Waited interminable hours, staring out windows blurring with rain and tears while Julie was examined and admitted.

Alone, I couldn't help Julie. Now I was handing her over to strangers. Could I trust them? What else could I do?

■ ■ ■

I pick her up from the outpatient day program. It's a year since her release. "Mummy," she sings out, "your little bunny ate all her dinner up. I had meatloaf and peaches and—oh, and Mummy, I'm making a teapot in ceramics with stars all over it."

■ ■ ■

Is it the pills talking, or the illness? Where is Julie?

And what happened in her last year at the private school? I'd heard rumours: bullying by staff, harassment from a fellow student, a date rape. Julie didn't talk. All I really know is, she went from being an asset to the school to being an embarrassment. Uninvited, she gave speeches in assembly denouncing the school system. She used exam time to compose a diatribe against teachers. She wandered the halls after lights out, wrote threatening notes, punched a girl in the back.

I cried over old photos of my once bright, smiling daughter, ready to conquer the world. Within a few months, Julie had undergone a complete personality change. At the staff's suggestion, we made several visits to the school psychologist. "It may be the onset of psychosis," he told me. "Only time will tell."

Her grades slipped but she graduated. When she came home to live, the real nightmare began. Emaciated, hollow-eyed, white-faced, with tangled black hair, black clothes, she disappeared for days at a time. She barely spoke. A few months later, she moved to Montreal, cut her ties with family and friends, moved in with Sunshine.

I couldn't reach her. Neither could anyone else. "Let her go," counsellors and social workers advised. "Back off. Don't interfere with her independence." Mothers were at worst meddlers and controllers, at best victims of the empty nest syndrome. There was nothing I could do, no help anywhere. Every night I wrapped myself in an old sweater she had left behind and, last thing before going to sleep, sent her a loving thought. I prayed that, in some indefinable way, it would reach her. I had to believe she felt my love.

■ ■ ■

Julie is lying in bed today, thumb in mouth. Nothing is working out. She wants to be a rock star but can't play the guitar, to be a baby so everyone will love her, to be crazy again so she won't have to clean her room. She wants to be Darlene on the Roseanne show.

■ ■ ■

Why this illness? Brain chemistry, one kindly doctor says. Not environment, nobody's fault. Stress, yes, but it was only a matter of time, the genes were there. Because of unusual determination, intelligence, and resilience, she was able to live a marginal existence in Montreal for two years before a complete psychotic break. Were there warning signs? Julie had always been somewhat unrealistic, obsessive. But weren't all children? At nine she wanted to be an Olympic figure skater, a ballerina, a champion gymnast. Isn't it part of growing up, being dazzled by the adult world, determined to do great deeds, to find some way to live forever? If Julie was more intense than some children, she was also more gifted. If she was more driven, wouldn't her passion find ways to channel itself into a productive, successful life?

I went every day to the hospital. Some days she lay with her face to the wall, groggy from the antipsychotic Haldol. Twice she sent me away. Usually, she met me with lists of things to buy: food, bottled water, vitamins, special moisturizer for her sensitive skin, special toothpaste for her tingling gums, special shampoo for her damaged hair. Pens, notebooks, labels, file cards. Her wall was covered with instructions, codes, cryptic warnings. She seesawed between eating voraciously and refusing everything except food from home, fearing the hospital fare was tainted. She made up a bed on the floor, rejecting the hospital cot. The staff humoured her. She ordered me to make her an eye appointment, not believing that blurred vision was a side effect of medication. She sent birthday cards to dozens of people—some she hardly knew—and invitations exhorting them all to come to Ottawa, spend Christmas at our house. "Is it wise to let her send mail?" I asked the staff. "When she's well again, she'll be embarrassed." "Patients' rights," they quoted.

Julie waited eagerly for the mail each day. Only one friend wrote.

On Haldol she paced endlessly, couldn't concentrate, thought her teeth were moving. University had started and she was frantic to be released. After a month, she refused the Haldol. The staff held her down and administered it by needle.

A switch to another antipsychotic, Stelazine, brought minimal improvement. Weekends she came home, made endless long distance calls, couldn't sit long enough to eat dinner. Once, she pulled me upstairs to hide under a bed: snipers were firing from a nearby rooftop.

The ward doctor withheld diagnosis, wavered between manic depression and schizophrenia. "She's schizophrenic—delusional, hallucinatory," staff members told me firmly. "Get a second opinion, don't waste time. There are new treatments. You want the best for her."

Another month elapsed before doctors conducting a schizophrenia study on the hospital's fifth floor prescribed a new antipsychotic, risperidone. Almost immediately, her symptoms abated.

After two full months, Julie came home on low doses of risperidone and the antidepressant Prozac. Anxious to resume activities in the outside world, still somewhat confused and barely able to focus, she pushed herself, entered a beauty contest, wrote a short story, signed up to sell Avon, made a video, took ceramics classes.

■ ■ ■

Today it's the shrew's turn to hold forth. "That's not what I want," Julie says as I come home with groceries. "I told you to get low-cal. And I won't use this cheap stuff on my hair." She throws a container on the floor. "Drive me to the drug store." "Take a bus," I say. "I won't! I hate buses!" She storms upstairs.

■ ■ ■

The house was a shambles, Julie's room so littered it was impossible to set foot in it without stepping on something. Julie wavered between tantrums and coy helplessness. She couldn't get her own breakfast, peel an orange, hang up her coat. She would spend hours organizing her pills but couldn't do laundry. If I got angry, she regressed. "Mummy doesn't love her little bunny," she cried. I walked a tightrope between being supportive and allowing myself to be manipulated.

■ ■ ■

Her brother drives up from Montreal for a weekend, bringing his new girlfriend. Julie can hardly wait to see Donnie, her favourite relative. We're so crowded they have to sleep in the living room, one on the sofa, one on the floor. Obstructing the TV just when Julie wants to watch a video. What promised to be a happy weekend turns into an ordeal, with taunting, accusing, vying for attention. "Mummy loves me better than she does you," she hurls at Donnie before flouncing off to her bedroom. "I don't want them here," she mumbles tearfully, thumb in mouth. "Mummy, please make them go home." They leave.

■ ■ ■

Finally unable to cope any longer, I went to her doctor. "It's a year since she was released," I said. "In all that time, I've had no help, no input from the hospital on how to live on a day-to-day basis. It could be just as valuable for you to know how things are at home, to help you administer to Julie's needs, as it would be for me to get advice from you."

The doctor leaned back and crossed his legs. "Julie has been very, very ill." As if I needed reminding.

"But what's my role? Her mood swings are bewildering, sometimes frightening. She frightens herself. It breaks my heart to see her like this."

"It's part of the illness."

"But is there no way she can control all this? It's as if when she's home she regresses to a time when she felt safe."

"She's not stabilized," the doctor pronounced. "We'll have to adjust her medication." Dismissed, I slunk away, the foolish, ignorant mother who had the temerity to approach a doctor and ask questions.

■　■　■

Julie and I sit in the doctor's office. "We're going to add lithium, a mood stabilizer," he says. "Keep taking risperidone and Prozac, keep up your salt intake. It'll take six weeks to start working. We test your blood twice weekly, to watch for toxicity." Julie's excited, wants to start it right away.

■　■　■

1994
She's been on risperidone a year, antidepressants almost as long. Now the doctor estimates a year for lithium. This fall Julie went back to university, commuting to Montreal two days a week. I'm not convinced that more medication is the answer. We take things a day at a time. She skates twice a week, good exercise and mental discipline. She concentrates on ice dancing, admitting, with some sadness, that she'll never be Oksana Baiul.

There is no solution. No recovered schizophrenics, just ways of controlling symptoms. There is no point in saying I should have done more. Acted sooner. Differently.

■ ■ ■

Julie creeps into my room at night, in her hearts-and-teddy-bears nightie. "Mummy, I love you best in the whole world." She clings to me for a long moment, and I hug her back.

■ ■ ■

We're going to get through this together, with love and patience and maybe this magic elixir, this formidable medicinal cocktail. We're raising Julie all over again, she and I together. Maybe we'll get it right this time.

Into the Bell Jar

Elm

SHANE NEILSON

> I know the bottom, she says. I know it with my
> great tap root:
> It is what you fear.
> I do not fear it: I have been there.
>
> —Sylvia Plath, "Elm"

At some point, I knew I was going mad. I knew, too, that the poetry was precipitating that descent. Yet I felt compelled, every evening, to tuck my daughter into bed and go into the basement office, where I'd hammer out poems about my alcoholic father and his eventual death. I wrote poems about his throwing me from the top mow of a barn, about his abuse of my mother. I kept going deeper and deeper into the story, the poetry getting darker and darker. *I kept getting darker and darker.*

I would go to work by day. At the start, work didn't suffer. I worked as a physician in the Emergency Department at the QEII hospital in Halifax, and I saw patients with efficiency. But as the poetic project unfolded, as one poem led to another, *I* began to suffer. Work began to suffer. I slowed down. I became critically unconfident. I repeated myself. I lost the thread of what patients were saying to me. Toward the end, patients were asking me, *Are you all right?*, having picked up on the fact that there was something wrong with their doctor.

I remember my last few patients: the fellow who had a self-inflicted gash across his wrist because "he just couldn't take it anymore," the guy who took a puck to the throat while watching a hockey game and who I had to intubate, a sixteen-year-old girl with abdominal pain and a positive pregnancy test, a horde of coughing people, a broken wrist, a dislocated shoulder, several lacerations, a drug overdose. I remember them all now, all very clearly.

As I treated these patients, I felt like I was wearing a rapidly fraying disguise. Before the start of every shift I would take a minute, inhale deeply, and mentally try to draw tight, to focus, to try to put on a mask that announced, *I'm here, I'm able.* To everyone, but especially to myself, I insisted: *yes, I'm all right.* I can continue working. When what I was really saying to myself was something quite different: *as long as I'm working, I'm fine.* I held on to that. It held on to me. It was part of my identity, my doctorhood. And for a time, the disguise held.

After a shift I would go home and clear the decks: attend to my daughter, who was three at the time, and spend time with my wife, who was aware that something was the matter but who felt powerless to do anything about it. I hurried through my husband and father role as quickly as possible in order to make time to write.

Then night would come, and I would go and write. Each night, there would be another poem. I wrote furiously, prolifically. I kept it up for a period of about three months, ending up with about a hundred poems, a dozen of which I would later keep. And each day I would wake up again, incrementally drained, and go back to work.

At one point I did wonder: is it the poetry that is doing this to me? Is it the poetry that's causing me to lose focus, to mumble, to contemplate my own death? I knew that there was something wrong with how I was thinking and feeling, and this bothered me, but not as much as it should have. I shrugged it off, saying to myself: well, I've been a poet for years. Poetry never hurt me before—quite the contrary. Poetry was the most life-affirming impulse I had at one point. Why should it hurt me now?

Oh, I don't know. Perhaps it was. During lulls in the process of writing about my father, I'd knock off little ditties like "Juncture":

> There is no emancipation
> in the stride off the chair,
> noose cinched about the neck;
> nor the bullet, with its instantaneous hammer.
> The exhaust pipe induces unpleasant cough,
> and wrists—veiny plains for melancholic settlers—
> are too compressible a crop,
> the red flow waning on pressed, anemic flesh.
>
> A drop to jump and hit the floor—
> in this, a real freedom. The plunge,
> a dive towards a bottoming,
> and the freefall, descent in pure vertical axis,
> a moment in suspension, and the bliss
> of stepping off, before the consequence;
> no swallowing of gunmetal shaft
> or the deliberation of knots.
> Only the urge of footsteps.
> Then air.

The thing was, I thought that this was just a poem, not a warning. There really is a point where one is beyond return, and, looking back, poems like "Juncture" practically scream this at me now.

■   ■   ■

The cycle of work and poetry repeated itself until, after what would be my last shift, I went to the basement one final time and wrote a poem about the death of my father, about his eventual demise as a result of falling from atop a tractor-trailer (he was a truck driver). I remember finishing the poem; I remember thinking, *I'm done. This is the last poem that is needed. I have finished.* Before I walked down there, I certainly had thoughts about my own death. I had been thinking about it more and more as time passed. I was sure that I wanted the death to have symmetry with my father's. I began to feel that it was inevitable, this death; but before I wrote that last poem, I had no idea it would be tonight.

I called up a blank screen and typed out:

> Goodbye. You're all better off without me. This is
> what I have to do and none of you are to blame.

I then walked up the stairs. It was about one o'clock in the morning; my wife and daughter were asleep, as usual. I left the laptop open on the kitchen counter and walked out onto the balcony.

It was a campaign of denial: sure, I thought about killing myself, but that seemed natural at the time. I couldn't hold a conversation with another person without shifting back to my own fractured thoughts, aimless and adrift. I couldn't read and comprehend, I couldn't study; I just wanted to be alone, and being alone meant writing. I lost forty pounds. I thought of life as unremitting pain. But could I pull it all together for one more shift in the Emergency Department? I thought I could.

One could see the neon lights from the nearby supermarket. There was no noise. It was cool and moist. I felt like I was doing something necessary, and that everyone would understand. I wasn't thinking of the certain bereavement of my family; I was thinking of certain release. I was thinking of the pain experienced to present, and of how, based on past experience, there would only be pain in the future. To die was to end the pain; to die was release.

I stepped over the railing. I was unafraid; it felt like the right thing to do. Without hesitation, I jumped.

■ ■ ■

I look back on this and wonder: how could I have thought so wrong? I had a beautiful wife, I had a healthy young daughter, I had a promising career, I was finding success as a writer. The explanation I have is one that was handed to me by my physicians who came to take care of me, that of the diagnosis of bipolar disorder. I must admit, my behaviour is inexplicable to me without that explanation. Yet, three years later, I'm left wondering: how much was it poetry's fault? How much did the poetry contribute to my deterioration? In the age of poetry as therapy, I went at things the opposite way: poetry as malady. The fact is that I wrote for hours a day, scrounging up a poem a day, and I got sicker with each one.

Now I'm sure the obvious retort here is that it was the *subject* that was the cause of my decline. It was revisiting the difficult past that was the problem, not the act of poetry itself. Yet I would say that I am a poet; I was a poet long before the jump, and as a poet what else could I be expected to write about? What else was as important? Wouldn't writing about bombs in Afghanistan be somehow dishonest without writing first about the explosions in my own childhood?

Then there is the matter of my work. But there, too, I had been a physician for years before getting sick, and there seemed nothing about the work itself that could contribute to madness. Sure, I was busy. Sure, it was stressful. But it had always been so. I enjoyed it. I felt much more ambivalent about the poetry I felt *compelled* to write; I never felt compelled to be in the Emergency Department.

■ ■ ■

Mad poets are nothing new. Wordsworth said it all in "Resolution and Independence" when he wrote, "We poets in our youth begin in gladness; but thereof comes in the end despondency and madness."

Poe, a renowned depressive, wrote "The Conqueror Worm," which speaks rather starkly about his mental state:

> But see, amid the mimic rout
> A crawling shape intrude!
> A blood-red thing that writhes from out
> The scenic solitude!
> It writhes!—it writhes!—with mortal pangs
> The mimes become its food,
> And the angels sob at vermin fangs
> In human gore imbued.

This wasn't merely a Poe grotesquerie; this was how he felt about the human endeavour. For her part, Sylvia Plath stuck her head in a gas oven after she had written the poems that transcend the sensationalism of her death. And Robert Lowell, my favourite poet, suffered cruel cycles of mania, and his poems are either the result of or in spite of his rather frightening manic depression. The list is inexhaustible. And for each, who can say whether the poetry contributed to their madness or whether they merely happened to be poets who were mad? It's impossible to know, and easy to speculate.

I don't even know in my own case.

In the hospital, when I was on one-to-one suicide watch, I wasn't allowed to write. It was felt that writing was a "trigger" for me, to use their parlance, and so it was outlawed. I spent a month not being able to go to the bathroom without the door opened a crack, I couldn't leave the hospital ward at all, I had no shoes for fear of elopement, I couldn't meet with my wife without a staff member also being present. Eventually the fear of suicide waned, and I was given more freedom. But I remained in the hospital for a further five months as various drugs were tried until one was found that was effective. Even when I was permitted to have a laptop, when I was able to write without fear of having nurses immediately read what I had written, I wrote no poems.

This is not to say that I didn't hear the same music, the same words calling to me, the snippets and phrases that present themselves to the poet who has his antennae up. I just didn't write them down, I didn't heed them. And I pointedly ignored them for three years.

Why? Well, I liken what happened to me to the experience one might get in a restaurant. Imagine eating a tainted piece of chicken and then spending days with bloody diarrhea, abdominal pain, fever, and vomiting. At the very least, one wouldn't order that same dish at the same restaurant, no? Probably, one wouldn't go back there at all. To take things further, one might not eat chicken ever again.

Well, I once wrote poetry. I fell ill. The poetry was in some way intrinsic to the illness. And now I don't write poetry. It's almost like an allergy: I was exposed to poetry, and now I've developed an immune response to it. If you're allergic to penicillin, you don't take penicillin. Or you might die.

Yet I had misgivings about still considering myself a poet, which I did, even though I didn't write poetry anymore. I felt like a charlatan. Doesn't a poet have to write poems?

■   ■   ■

The thing illness robs us of, mental illness most of all, is perspective: we never really apprehend how sick we are until it's either too late or until we get well again and realize just how powerfully rendered we were, how vulnerable we were, how near death. Even poetry was perverted by my illness—what once was sense-making, and feeling-divining, came to seek a kind of banishment. I wrote poems to survive, I always had, and my illness took control of what was best in me. At my sickest I wrote poems presaging death, as death wishes, and ultimately they became a death act.

It's been many years since that jump from the balcony. I've returned to writing poems, and found some success. I fought fire with fire in my first book and wrote some poems about mental illness itself. Those were the most difficult poems I've ever written, and when I read them to audiences, as I sometimes do, I feel more than naked: I feel as if I am actually disappearing. I am also reminded, as I am sure I am supposed to be reminded, that I nearly died, and that if I am not careful, I may die again. This is the ultimate victory of poetry over the illness. It is a testament to survival.

I've built on the first book with a second that uses the practice of medicine as its theme; the greatest rumination of "Complete Physical" is, *How do we get well?* Poem after poem asks the same question, in sestinas, in sonnets, in villanelles, in lyrics, in narratives. And the answer is the same answer everyone breathes, and wakes up with, and goes to sleep to every day: we live because the pain does not define us. Philip Larkin wrote in "An Arundel Tomb" that "What will survive of us is love" and the problem of mental illness is that love is a higher-order emotion, one that we are deprived of when ill. On that balcony, I had no true accounting of how much love was being received or given. Years later, I know what was being forsaken.

But I have been on the balcony. I no longer fear it, for there have been poems about beauty too, about my wife and daughter and all the love I can ever carry. I'm still writing them, little anti-Elms. All the poems since are steps away from that precipice.

Over and Overcoming

YAHO-HANAN FIWCHUK

I suppose my most dramatic experience as a psychotic individual occurred a couple of months after my first encounter with the nether world—a voice coming from a Waterloo closet in the winter of 1983. I was twenty-four years old and enrolled in my third year of fine arts at the University of Waterloo.

I grew up near a paper mill in the small Ontario community of Thorold. The town is between Lake Erie and Lake Ontario, and the Welland Canal runs through it. My family was a hockey family headed by a father who believed in hard work. I didn't like to play hockey and had *problems* as a child. I wasn't a very happy kid.

To me Waterloo was a big place, but over the summer and fall of 1982 I began to focus on going to an even bigger place, New York City. I wanted to live life there as a painter. I practised getting to New York by walking on the train tracks near my residence on John Street. I walked aimlessly, not keeping track of time, often gone for whole afternoons. I moved from tie to tie, sometimes landing on the stones between. The tracks were ugly and desolate, and wound through a brewery, but I was comfortable because I was isolated.

At the time, I had stopped looking people in the eye—things

had begun to look threatening in my periphery. I felt menaced and paranoid. Eventually, in January 1983, I began to take direction from the voices. I believed the voices would get me to New York. I trusted they would tell me to "stay" when I was on the right track, or to turn right or left if need be.

My beloved paintings became fodder for destruction. I ripped all the canvases from the wooden stretchers and sawed everything into pieces. I made a pile of destroyed art three to four feet high in the middle of my bedroom. When I was finished sawing, I left it all behind and was ready to head out for New York City.

■ ■ ■

The first week of February, I began the journey down the tracks dressed in a bomber jacket with an overcoat overtop. For three days and nights I stayed outside, sleeping in snowbanks and eating nothing but the snow at the side of the tracks. All the while I was receiving messages from *spirits* telling me of my progress. "You're doing fine. Everything is taken care of." Sometimes I received signals—"Destultify yourself." I was mystified by these signals. While I walked, I tried to figure out what they meant. Occasionally the spirits told me to get off the tracks and walk on country roads, and eventually they told me to walk on a massive highway.

In Orangeville, about sixty kilometres from where I started, the cops picked me up and took me to some sort of hostel-hotel. I ate my first meal since leaving Waterloo and had a chance to dry my clothes, which had been soaked by the freezing rain that fell that night. Someone called my older sister to come and pick me up, but by the time she arrived I'd taken off again, heading toward Toronto. For years after that, she worried every night whether I had a safe place to sleep.

The next day while I was hitchhiking outside Toronto—on what I think by the size of it must have been Highway 401—a Catholic priest pulled over onto the shoulder. He picked me up and drove me to the Sally Ann, where they gave me a hot meal and a bed. I had been walking so much and had been wearing such crappy hiking boots, thick chunks of flesh fell off my feet when I took the boots off to try to sleep. But the spirits started talking to me again. They told me, "Get up. Get dressed." I hit the streets again.

That night, a souped-up Chevy Nova with wide Mag wheels was stopped for speeding right in front of me. The driver was out of his car talking with the cop when a voice said, "Take the car." So I did. While I drove down the Don Valley Expressway, the voices told me the cars beside me had demons in them and I must "knock them off the road."

Eventually the Nova swerved, hit the guardrail, and came to a stop. Luckily no one was hurt; that is, until I was arrested. The cop who pulled me out of the Nova hit me while I was in the back of his car. I fell down onto the seat to avoid being hit again, but I was at peace because the voices said, "Everything is as planned." I ended up in a detective's office and from there went to the Don Jail in Toronto, where I was housed with all the castaways for whom no one cares.

■ ■ ■

After what felt like a long time, I went before a judge. My court-appointed lawyer told me I had to straighten up, which I managed to do somewhat. Then it was back to jail for I don't know how long before someone told me I should be at Met Fors (Metropolitan Forensics).

Met Fors was part of the Queen Street Mental Institute in Toronto, and it was the first place I received any medication. Trilafon made my tongue curl back so badly I had to bite on a towel to keep myself from swallowing my tongue. Still the voices did not dissipate. I remember sitting in a room there with my parents and asking them if they heard the voices. Ultimately I figured out I was alone in this. But Met Fors was very clean and I felt safe. I don't remember much else about my time there except the people were kind. I don't think they ever did figure me out.

■ ■ ■

In April of that year, I was released, given a few dollars, a bail of Daily Mail institutional tobacco, and a referral to the John Howard Society. I was told they would give me a job to keep myself busy, but they weren't much help and I wasn't able to work anyway. I needed social assistance. I couldn't hold a job. It was my first time in a big city. Everything was pretty much broken up.

I walked around during the day for something to do. At night, I slept at the Sherbourne Street Sally Ann, notorious for vagrants. There were a dozen or so rooms set up as little dorms, each with at least six beds. In total, seventy to eighty people slept there, all of them men. Twice a week we lined up to get a ticket: one punch was good for a night and three punches was good for a day of meals.

Every morning we were kicked out of bed at 7:00 AM, and we went around back, into the basement, to get toast, a hardboiled egg (I kept mine in my pocket), and oatmeal. Coffee was in a pail on the floor with a ladle to fill a melamine cup. We could come back to the basement for lunch and dinner but had to leave after each meal and not come back until 7:00 PM, when we could get into the dorm.

I remember the first lunch I ate was some kind of pink slop with beans and vegetables. Another man watching me said, "That guy actually ate two plates."

Only one night did I miss the 11:00 PM curfew. I tried to sleep on a bench in Queen's Park, but there were too many strange people walking around. I ended up at an all-night coffee shop with a friend, but we only had money enough for one coffee so we nursed it all night long.

■ ■ ■

In August of that year, I found out it didn't snow in Vancouver. I began working part-time to earn the money to buy a bus ticket. Ninety-nine bucks would get you anywhere in Canada on the bus in those days. Early every morning, I went down to the corner of Queen and Sherbourne, to a bay at the back of a warehouse, where a guy called out, "You. You and You." He'd buy those of us he'd picked a breakfast, take it off our pay, and load us into a truck. We were driven to Mississauga, where we delivered flyers through a long day.

By the end of September, I had saved enough to buy a ticket to Vancouver. I arrived the first week of October and it rained for three weeks—my nose ran the whole time. But I found places to live in the West End and in Kitsilano. For a time I stayed at the Barclay Manor, which had the street name of Bad Manners, but I never landed in the Downtown Eastside and for that I am grateful.

The whole time I had been waiting to get back to art. Eventually in 1985, I got myself organized enough to enroll at the University of British Columbia, again in the fine arts program. I wanted to finish my degree but found there were too many distractions and I couldn't concentrate. There also seemed to be too much red tape around transferring my credits from the University of Waterloo to UBC. All I could do was paint, and nothing else. I became discouraged and quit.

During this time, I was on and off medications. Some of them made the skin around my nose crack badly, some made my legs cycle as if I were riding a phantom bicycle. I still did not take my illness seriously.

One day in the fall of 1986, I was down in Chinatown looking for my Uncle Nick. I asked around for him and people told me to look for the black Corvette—that he lived above where I would find it parked. I found the Corvette and my Uncle Nick somewhere near East Pender or Cordova. He took me to my first meeting at the Assembly of Yahowah the Eternal. My uncle normally didn't smile much, and he was not a regular attender, but he told me about the assembly with such joy in his voice and animation in his body, I decided to check it out.

The first time I went to the assembly was in January 1987. The people were warm and friendly, and I could see they were searching for the truth. Together with them, I began to use the major religious texts and guides—the Bible, the Torah, the Koran, *The*

Tibetan Book of the Dead—to find the truths that can be proved. I was told Yahowah was not going to come down and heal my schizophrenia, but that he is near all of us and could guide me physically and spiritually.

The truths of the assembly can be difficult to discern, and perhaps for too long a time I believed that Yahowah would be offended by my painting. With that fear and the words of my father in my head—"You'll die and the rich will inherit your paintings"—I threw all of my art into a dumpster in 1987. I didn't paint for twenty years, until 2007 when one morning I woke up and thought to myself, *I feel like painting again*. Also at that time my best friend Gordon had passed away, and painting gave me a platform to express my emotions and thoughts.

But despite my confusion over whether to paint or not, the assembly helped me with my situation and I began to find the strength to deal with my illness. It wasn't until I accepted the fact that I was sick that I started to get better. Through the assembly I learned to meditate, and I read many learned philosophical pieces. *The Tibetan Book of the Dead* talks about "bringing it all home," and when I feel myself becoming psychotic I use the teachings and meditation to bring it all to a point so I can let it go. I repeat to myself, "Bring it all home." Then when it comes to a point, I tell myself, "Release. Relax."

■　■　■

I know I am becoming psychotic when I hate my own flesh, when I question everything and no one has answers, when everything around me seems negative and I can't let it go, can't go with the flow, even the air becomes an enemy (while I watch the world around me decay).

Thoughts swirl—reality is hard to find—everything seems to bear down on me. So I get changed into some clean cotton sleep apparel, and some clean cotton sheets, and I wrap up in a bed cocoon, and focus on the ugly until I can bring it down to a small kernel that can be set aside. I like the winter so I can make the cocoon. In summer I lie on top of the bed with a sheet and try to keep myself below all the thoughts above me. If I don't have the time to get home, I will just close my eyes no matter where I am—in a restaurant, at the assembly—and try to bring everything to a point and calm down.

The episodes can be painful and often hit in the late afternoons. They are difficult to describe, but it starts as an agitation in the periphery. I feel menaced and threatened, want to disconnect. I know it's a brain activity, and if I can get hold of it and release it in time, the activity will clear quickly. Other times it can take twenty minutes, sometimes hours.

My ailing health has been bothersome to date, but I consider myself an overcomer—over and over again. When I become psychotic, I *Lone Ranger* it until it passes. It always passes, at least that's what I tell myself (with a handful of multicoloured pills). Every day I take more than twenty pills. Lithium, risperidone, Loxapine, Seroquel, Ativan as needed, and vitamins including niacin and B-complex. I like learning new things using my mind and my body. I study philosophy, and I study tai chi. But it can be hard with the pills—like being stoned. Now that I have an acute awareness of my illness, I have a great deal more peace of mind. I have no more dangerous thoughts or actions, and no more voices, although I still have some frightening associations triggered by sounds. Sometimes I'll be in heavy traffic or a large crowd and it will seem like a collective force is coming against me. When I am doing well, I can be in the same situation and hear the same noises and it does not affect me. One regret I have is that after years of treatment, I don't feel as connected to the earth as I used to. Maybe I'm just getting older.

But I take the bull's horns and there I pray and deal with this illness of mind—my affliction. Something so personal, a few words on paper do it no justice. So I paint. Moving colour on canvas does the job, oh so well.

My soul is left imprinted on confines of not more than 20" x 20" (that's all my easel will hold). But what I see is not the truth, only an abstract extension of internal plight. The apartment where I live is full with my paintings and sketchbooks.

■　■　■

My life is one of recurring themes—cycles and patterns—some days go very slowly and are very painful; all I want to do is get into bed and shut if off. But most days, I get up, take a walk, do some errands, paint for two to five hours, sometimes cradling the canvas in my arm like a violin, and I listen to Dylan—he's so inspiring to paint by. I organize art shows and I make plans like everyone else. Like John Lennon said, "Life is what happens to you while you're busy making other plans."

The paintings reflect. Time is a friend. Pain is time's sister. Reality looms. And I say g'night.

Atlas & the Cheese Cube

CATHERINE OWEN

Nibbles: an introduction

It is the fall of 1991. I am at the Vancouver International Writers
Festival, nineteen years old and thrilled by my very first Poetry
Bash whose line-up includes Susan Musgrave, Patrick Lane, and
esteemed American poet Sharon Olds. After the gala, some of my
friends wander into the backstage area to chat with the poets; I,
nervous, hang back. Before long, one of them returns with a story
that eventually means more to me than I understand at the time.
My friend had been talking to Sharon Olds at one of the folding
tables the organizers had set up behind the curtained-off podium.
The poet, amid her repartee, had kept arranging and rearranging
the square crackers and cheese cubes she had placed on her paper
plate. She seemed unable to eat them, perhaps stymied by the
conversation from being able to organize the nibbles in a way that
appeared aesthetically "right" to her. Her anxiety appeared to rise as
they spoke, her hands preoccupied by the need to structure her food
prior to eating it.

My friend was bemused and a little confused as she relayed
this tale to me, tossing out "Total OCD," as if it was a punchline

to a joke. This was the first time I had heard the condition spoken of, however spuriously, in public. Connecting Olds's compulsion to obsessively arrange her aperitifs in a "safe" mode with my own experience of the disorder not only made me feel closer to my favourite poet of the day, but valorized in some way the likelihood that I could live a vital, if somewhat circumscribed, life as an artist despite my equivalent craving for repetition and my similar need for a grounding in visual and aural certainties.

While many who don't understand obsessive compulsive disorder (OCD) tend to dismiss it with such statements like, "I think about stuff a lot too" or "You're such a neat freak," those who truly suffer from the condition find that OCD patterns and behaviours consume a large part of their daily activities or thoughts. Living with OCD can be like existing in a continually twisting kaleidoscope in which one cannot just let the bits fall as they may. One must strain always to master their tumblings, to replicate their structures, to keep breathing despite the wilfulness of all those fragments in their relentless descent.

Not one drop of oil, not one speck of dirt: my father and OCPD

My father is the third child of four and the youngest son. As a sensitive, artistic, philosophically minded young man of twenty, he met my British-born, thirty-one-year-old mother at a gathering in Vancouver in 1969 and they were married ten months later. She had left the convent two years prior, deeply desiring a family after spending more than a dozen years as a nun. My fully-in-love father, disillusioned with his university studies and wanting children too, was in agreement. I arrived in 1971, and he became the conflicted and perfectionistic truck driver he remains, father to five, now grandfather to eleven, still living with my mother in the unique front and back duplex he built in Burnaby.

Along with being raised in the light of my father's interests in literature, culture, religion, and current events, I also grew up in the shadow of his obsessive compulsive personality disorder (OCPD). While someone with OCD can spend hours lining up the coffee mugs, scrubbing the same spot on the counter over and over again, or checking if the door is locked countless times before being able to leave the house, the person with OCPD will obsess about keeping the house clean to prevent disease or display compulsions that include recycling, composting, or other activities that aim to reduce waste. They are hoarders but always for a stated purpose; they are repeaters but always to attain a particular end. As rigid leaders, they reign supreme over what they think must be accomplished and have little capacity or desire to yield to the collaborations of others. Their obsessions and compulsions appear logical, necessary, simply the "right" way to do things, but they nonetheless take such actions to the extreme. My father, otherwise one of the noblest, most generous, and most intelligent men I know, has a condition that, at its most intense, turns him painfully irritable, aggravating. In such moments, I can scarcely bear to be near him.

The kitchen has always been the focal room for his disorder. While my mother, who remained a homemaker throughout our childhoods, cooked the evening meal, my father's department appeared to be everything else that occurred there. His OCPD demanded that he domineer over most areas from food preparation to clean up. My clearest impression of all those years of OCPD flare-ups was of myself as a highly fallible mouse scuttling about beneath the dangerous gaze of an ever-watchful hawk, albeit one in Dickies pants and rubber gloves, who might pounce at any moment with admonishments or anger. My siblings and I were told about "the method" of doing dishes, stirring the peanut butter, setting the table, flattening tin cans, tearing off lettuce leaves, but invariably, as we were not taught patiently how to do these things, and instead hectored about not doing them correctly, we never quite got it. There was always more than an inch of water in the sink, a drip of oil would run treacherously down the peanut butter jar, we cut our bread or tomatoes too thick on one side, too thin on the other, or we disrupted the visual balance of the dinner table by putting a squeeze bottle of ketchup on it.

These errors and more were destined to piss him off thoroughly, causing him to raise his voice, or jump up and grab the offending item from our hands, often muttering, "Stupid, stupid" as he undertook the job himself, all of us plainly incapable of the simplest tasks without creating waste or dirt or introducing a criminally unaesthetic element into the pure domestic picture. While his OCPD has lessened over the years, due either to wisdom or exhaustion, being reared in an environment where standards were impossible to achieve has rooted a case of the nerves in me when I get anywhere near a kitchen. Whether he's present or not, I am relentlessly failing to fulfill his methods and thus, in my mind's eye, am always being neglectful, slovenly, wasteful, or clumsy, a domestic wreck. It is not his fault, this mental illness. And yet, neither has he sought help for this condition. It's always been: "You know what your father's like."

Tap, tap, tap, tap: a brief interlude on my son and OCD

My son wants to tell his own story of a life lived under the sometimes oppressive and occasionally inspirational hand of OCD and someday he will. Born when I was sixteen, my son likely developed OCD following my divorce from his father, when he was five years old. He struggled throughout his childhood with two central types of OCD: touching and intrusive thoughts, the initial one developing first and later linking mysteriously with the latter. Tapping objects in patterns partially helped him to define the parameters of his often-chaotic existence; at the same time this urge interrupted schoolwork, entertainment, personal relationships, and could occasionally be dangerous. Around the age of seven, he became convinced his eyes were capable of "leaping out" in the direction of whatever his gaze fell upon. Thus, when he looked at anything, even if it was in the middle of the road, he would run to retrieve his "eyes." Once he'd fetched them, he then needed to "paste" them back in his face with a predictable pattern of taps. If he felt incapable of acting on this impulse, he would become saddened, even enraged.

As he became an adolescent, it was unwanted thoughts about everything from illness to rape that swarmed through his mind, unbearable obsessions that made him cry, scream, or even threaten to hurt himself. He went to several psychiatrists over a period of ten or so years but has never responded well to pharmaceuticals. Now in his early twenties, he has begun to surmount his turmoil more successfully, but the struggle never entirely sleeps. To control his compulsions, he has tried meditation, yoga, Reiki, and shifting his obsessiveness to a passion for cooking; for a period of time, he also took medical marijuana. And yet, sadly, I often feel anxious or nervous around him, steeling myself against his outbreaks of obsessive thoughts, their spillage poisoning our difficult, demanding, yet often amazingly enriching bond. In my father, I see the essential conditions for the development of my own OCD; in my son, I witness the repercussions of this mental illness and the frightening array of faces this Hydra-headed condition can display.

Three Little Cowboys in a Row: My experience of OCD

The earliest memory I have of my own OCD is benign, yet it reveals the central shape this illness was to take in my life: it would not surround cleaning or praying or counting but ordering and its underlying principles of balance, equality, and control. I was six years old, attending my aunt's wedding, feeling both fancy and out of sorts in a dress and shiny shoes, sitting in the pew with my sisters and another uncle, who leaned over to me halfway through the ceremony and whispered, "I see you've finally got all that perfect then," his eyes twinkling at me and my quaint preoccupation. I had been arranging and rearranging my corsage spray between the hymnals throughout the length of the service. Even then I sought both aesthetic and psychological harmony. Yet I grew self-conscious after my uncle pointed out my behaviour, and I asked myself why others at the ceremony didn't feel the need to perform such rituals; how were they content to let their hymnals sit crookedly, to just toss their flowers willy-nilly on the seat beside them, never even glancing once at the bouquet to see if it had retained its position or if it needed to be shifted slightly one inch to the left or right?

Becoming aware of this personality trait didn't stop these preoccupations, it merely increased my sense of difference from others, my isolation. I tried not to perform my ritualistic orderings in public, attempting instead to silence these impulses with ritual manners of dress. I would sport an equal number of coloured elastic bands on each wrist, for example, and when I grew anxious in my urge to publicly order things I would refer this ache to my elastic bands, quietly taking them off and putting them on again according to colour and number until I felt calmer, more self-contained. I had my own room from the time I was in grade one and it became my OCD haven. Fortunately I was smart enough to excel in school, considering I spent an exorbitant amount of time involved in obsessive "hobbies" like pulling all my books out of the bookcase by approximately two inches and then pushing them back against the wall again, in a row from the left end to the right, until I had heard each text make its satisfying click against the plaster. Other days I would line up one of my collections to linear perfection, adjusting my hoards of Tic Tac boxes, animal figurines, or plastic Cowboy and Indian models until they formed a satisfying row on my windowsill. When I couldn't arrange my small world, I would take refuge in becoming ill. Incapable of functioning in public during the time that my coping mechanisms had faltered, I would spend days beneath the sheets, suffering from a weird range of conditions, like reflex sympathetic dystrophy, an illness that made my limbs cold, stiff, and blue.

By the time I reached my teens, I had started to spend hours in front of the mirror, mostly an odd little vanity glass I had in my room whose surface could shift from yellow to pink to blue light at the touch of a switch. I would nudge this toggle slowly from left to right and, as the light altered its shades, examine my face for pimples, excess hair, freckles, or any other perceived flaw. I would do the same to my body, deeming it too skinny, too flat. I was horribly self-conscious about being looked at too closely and especially of a boy commenting on my physical failings. One absurd memory stands out in particular. I had gone to an ultimate football game with a grade ten boyfriend and, on using the washroom prior to the start of the match, had spied a pimple on my chin, even worse, it was an off-centred pimple and marred, I thought, my entire face. There followed a long period, it might have been up to an hour, where I tried to burst the pimple or, failing that, to conceal it with cover-up. I undertook each attempt so many times, becoming increasingly sickened with my obsessiveness to the point of nausea, sweats, and weakness, that I not only created a suppurating wound on my chin that would leave a scar but I made myself so ill trying to attain impossible perfection that I fainted. I awoke in the medics' room at BC Place, my boyfriend fussing confusedly over me. I was humiliated, despairing at the extremes my condition had taken me to.

Getting pregnant in my mid-teens, after a period of promiscuity undertaken partly to allay my fears of being ugly and thus undesirable, only gave my OCD more inadequacies to feed on as the mirror sessions extended to changes in my physique caused by pregnancy and breastfeeding. Now, in my late thirties, my OCD, as expressed through this body dysmorphia, tends to focus more on wrinkles rather than pimples. Fortunately, over the years I've become so accustomed to the "voices" of OCD that I am often successful at removing myself from the sources of its torment, whether the mirror or an especially critical individual, before I dismantle my self-esteem.

Where I continue to struggle is with the way that OCD has internalized itself linguistically. No longer so obsessed with controlling the external world (though lint on a black carpet will invariably drive me crazy), I now have to repeat certain word combinations or phrases in my head before I can accomplish the actions they refer to. For instance, I might recite silently, "Now I'll read, write, and study." I can never just say, "Now I'll read a book," or repeat nothing at all before settling down with a novel. The pattern must occur in threes, must contain a certain number of syllables, must be aurally balanced. I also have set statements that I repeat mentally on a regular basis. One of these is "in every way, shape, and form." So I might recite, "I have to shower, shampoo, and shave in every way, shape, and form." Additionally, I also have "hinge" or "short-cut" words that I tack on to many thoughts. One of these is the neologism "multiplicitous," and I use it to encompass everything I can't list in the moment, thinking for instance, "today I am doing multiplicitous activities." These phrases and words are entirely unnecessary for sense, completely essential for my OCD.

Much of what I plan to do must be listed, sometimes on paper and more often within my head before it can be accomplished. If the list promises to be too lengthy, unwieldy, and full of messy bits of sound, I avoid the activity connected to this task. For instance, I will steer clear of smorgasbords or buffets because I have to list all the food items in my head prior to consuming them. So I will only eat "toast and yogourt and coffee" in the morning, the three types of food with their resonant "o" sounds enabling me to swallow them, whereas if I were faced with a meal of multiple dishes my mind would be far too preoccupied with the required listing to consume a morsel. Conversing can also be a torment to me. My words, incapable of arranging themselves in prior fashion, are likely to emerge imperfectly, a situation that can create intense frustration for me and the desire to avoid off-the-cuff opportunities in order to spare myself this stress.

Although I'm an accomplished writer who has two degrees, the consuming nature of my OCD has impeded relationships and jobs. I am opposed to pharmaceuticals and have never found psychiatrists particularly helpful in the treatment of this condition, preferring to use self-talk in order to overcome some of its more debilitating manifestations. Whether I like it or not, however, in the end I deal with my OCD by spending perhaps more time alone than most people. I toil in the realm of lists, working to ensure balance within myself and to endure the out-of-control feeling that overcomes me when I just can't "get it right" no matter how many sounds I place, just so, side by side by side.

Bipolar Babe

ANDREA PAQUETTE

I believed the earth was shaking when I was first in the psych ward, when actually a snow blower had come up against the window causing my adrenalin levels to rise in terror. Another patient ran to my side, assuring me that I was okay, but I was not convinced. I hid in the pitch-black laundry room thinking it was the only safe place in the hospital, and in the next heartbeat I thought I would be crushed to death by a pending earthquake. I had to keep moving, even if it was in circles, around and around the ward.

I walked the hallways, unable to sleep for days, ingesting pill after pill, trying to close my eyes, which felt spry and stapled open. When I observed my reflection in the mirror I saw something divine. I believed my body was a holy temple for souls to rest in. But despite my intense spiritual experiences, I just continued walking the hallways, unable to sleep.

I was only twenty-six years old and I was being hospitalized for the second time. I will never forget my new psychiatrist first approaching me and asking if I was okay. Earlier that day I had felt beaten to a pulp, but when he spoke I was listening to the gentlest and kindest voice I had heard in years. My previous doctor, at the other end of the country in Ottawa, was also magnificent—a gentle French man—but his office was bright yellow and I believed the colour stimulated my hunger (perhaps explaining my thirty-five-pound weight gain). But this new doctor, Dr. J, seemed to care even more whether I was okay. He told me I should take a shower, something I had not done for days, and I was motivated to do it.

Dr. J reminded me of how special and successful I was. Even after I had been out of the hospital for only a couple of weeks, and even though I had met him because of a suicide attempt and he had prescribed me six months of medication, he never questioned me. Not even when I was determined to go to Korea to teach English. He trusted and respected me. This was amazing because I never respected myself.

When I rambled on about creating an organization about bipolar disorder, he never seemed to doubt me. And now I see his pride when he invites his students to sit in on my sessions. I imagine them chatting after I leave about how intelligent, successful, and driven I am, or at least I hope they do, and this makes me proud.

Why do I constantly need others to reinforce in me what I ought to already know myself? The stigma associated with mental illness implies that people who have one are unintelligent, and I seem to believe it as I constantly seek reinforcement from Dr. J, my boyfriend, my case manager, and my family and friends. I feel like a hypocrite. Should I not know this—that I *am* intelligent?

To help with the stigma, I began creating the project called Bipolar Babe. Now we are an army of survivors alongside others who want the survivors to survive. As I stare at the project's famous pink logo with the tough little superhero squishing the word *stigma*, I am reminded how important it is to create conversations free of stigma, especially with our youth, who are still forming their own opinions with their open and blossoming minds.

One aspect of the project entails speaking in classrooms and sharing my personal experience. I question concepts such as madness, mental illness, and mental distress, and my hope is to create acceptance and understanding among all kids, to ensure that nobody suffers in silence. Our Bipolar Babe team on Vancouver Island has hosted the successful Bipolar Babe Benefit: Hair Show and Art Gala, and in front of a large crowd, I have shared my experience of having bipolar disorder. It feels as comfortable as having a conversation with my best friend. Yet, there was a time not long ago that I could barely look at myself in the mirror and be comfortable admitting that I had bipolar disorder.

I also recently created the Bipolar Disorder Society of BC alongside five other founding directors. Now that I have arrived in this place, it feels like I have reached the most significant milestone of my life. I have raved about the project on numerous radio shows and each time it feels like I get a little piece of my heart back. It reminds me that all the pain and torture I went through was somehow significant and meaningful. Now I can share it with the world and I can finally heal. Though sometimes I still wonder, When does the healing begin and where does it end?

I remember in the fall of 2007, I was crying to Dr. J about the drug abuse and the callous way that I had treated myself. It was at this time that I decided to stop drinking alcohol and cease all substance abuse. He and my case manager listened intently and he wrote quickly to keep up with my tears. It was from that day forward that I changed my life. Rehab was mentioned, but instead I created my own solace. I soon became reclusive but in a healthy way, surviving on phone calls, DVDs, and my computer to keep me sane.

If Dr. J had not entered my life, where would I be today? I have no clue. Although I do not owe my life to him, I hear of the horror stories of other psychiatrists' relationships with their patients and I recognize how fortunate I am. They don't have a relationship. Dr. J knows people and knows how to have relationships. Being under his care has helped me to create a type of safety system, which I call my mental health security net. Now I am able to teach others that they, too, can play an active role in their health and weave this net by aiming to secure a medical team and do their part in developing a reciprocal and respectful relationship. I encourage people with a mental illness to spend time educating themselves and share their personal experience of having a mental illness with family and friends. I have found it helpful to be honest with my employer to ensure that my place of employment is supportive, especially if I have to miss work due to my illness. It's also been useful to link into the services in my local mental health community and participate in support groups. A healthy diet is important, and plenty of water flushes the medication through my system, ensuring optimal performance. I always try to get adequate sleep, and I have realized how vital it is to have the sunshine on my face especially on long walks by myself or with a loved one. I am assured that with this recipe if I ever were to fall, I would surely be caught.

Having bipolar disorder means I have floated so high I have literally seen the stars below me in a breathtaking gaze above the earth. And in the next heartbeat, I have seen the devil's face dance and laugh at me during a torrid and insane psychosis. It feels as real as breathing air into my lungs, and as natural as opening my eyes when I wake in the morning. Bipolar affective disorder has brought me to my knees, made me lose all ability to prepare a meal. And even when I do, I am unable to taste my food. *All* things become stale and bland. Taking a shower is as difficult as building an entire house. I become disabled and confined to my bed for days at a time.

However, bipolar illness has made me laugh harder, feel deeper, and at times made my thoughts flow in perfect harmony, allowing my creative juices to boil for poetry, art, and writing. Although my hands shake and I depend on medication to function, I see bipolar disorder as my cursed gift. It has brought me to open a space, a place where others can heal and share their story, and for this I am grateful.

Committed

ADDY S. PARKER

I meet with my manager, Mark, in his office. It's my regular weekly one on one that helps Mark keep track of what I'm working on and gives me a chance to ask for help if I need it. I never miss these meetings. The skills I need to navigate the corporate world I learned from the time I spent at the Brookview Adolescent Treatment Centre, or the Batty Centre, as the residents affectionately knew it. Weekly check-ins are important if you want people to see the effort you are putting in and the progress you are making.

I sit on the small beige sofa he bought at IKEA and pick at the wire binding of the spiral notebook in my lap. He looks at me, scratches his closely trimmed beard, and asks, "How are things going?" And then he continues typing on his computer keyboard.

"Okay." I focus out the window behind him, on the blue glass wall of the next wing of the building. I can see the square white lights of other computer monitors through the glare but none of the people. There's a company-sanctioned word for my mood. To my therapist, I might say that I am feeling overwhelmed and hopeless, and that I am having trouble concentrating. I might add that I have lost interest in activities that I used to enjoy. The corporate world has its own lexicon to describe problems in a way that relates to my professional commitments. "I guess the problem is that I'm just really"—I look up at the pinholes speckled about the ceiling tiles—"randomized right now."

In the early 1980s, when I was a child playing with BASIC on my TI-99 computer, I learned how to use a randomizing function. When run, the script would slowly fill the black monitor screen with a fuzz of different-coloured pixels—like mould growth recorded on time-lapse video. It would make my eyes mush and lose focus. Whenever I use the corporate phrase "I'm feeling randomized," I see this polychromatic moss and sense it spreading over me. It wraps around my throat and suffocates me. Randomization is depression dressed in business casual.

"Do you need help?" Mark jostles and clicks the mouse on his desk repeatedly. The screen's light flickers across his pupils. "Are you going to need help to meet your deadlines?"

"No." My problem is not one of adequate time but of adequate will. I'm bipolar and feeling a bit depressed this week. Someone poking around asking how they can help me is only going to force me to expend the last of my energy covering up the truth about me and about my unfinished work. "I just have to sit down and reprioritize. There are some things that don't have to be done until next month, I just haven't taken the time to sit down and schedule them all out. I'll do that now."

"Okay." Mark's chair creaks mechanically like an emergency brake as he leans back, pushing against the armrests to eke out a slight angle of recline. "Let me know if you need any help. I'm sure there will be someone on the team who has some free cycles."

"Thanks, Mark." I feel suddenly embarrassed by the direct eye contact. Although he doesn't know it, I'm the one with free cycles. I haven't done any real work for weeks. I clutch my notebook to my chest and lift myself up off the couch and out the door.

In my office, I log on to my computer and check all of my favourite blogs and web comics while I wait for five o'clock to roll around. All I can do is hope for a hypomanic spell to hit me before my deadlines come up. I can get a lot done in just a week of mood buzz. Too much, actually. When I'm emotionally high, I'm ambitious and fearless. I take on new projects, I innovate, I think big, I hardly sleep, I take risks. I make myself noticed, and I have a reputation as a hot shot on the team. When I'm depressed, I know how to make myself invisible and not detract from that reputation. The weeks of inactivity and flurries of productivity even out in the end and may even give me a slight advantage over my even-paced colleagues because, at least some of the time, I'm flashy.

When the hypomania is over, I'm left in a swamp of debts again. All those projects started and not finished, all those risks panning out or not, all that sleep lost, the money spent impulsively. When I come back down, it feels like I've been possessed by something that walked around in my skin getting me into all sorts of trouble that I can't explain because people will think I'm crazy.

But I need the high, or have come to need it. It's like the Hulk. And since I started turning into the Hulk, I find myself in situations I need the Hulk to get out of. Yet they are situations I wouldn't be in if the Hulk didn't exist in the first place. I'll be sitting at my desk late at night trying to finish the report I promised to have done by the end of the week, drinking Mountain Dew to stay awake and taking breaks to cry the fatigue out of my body. It may not even be possible for me to finish the report; there may be numbers I need that haven't even come in yet. That didn't bother the Hulk when she made the schedule because she knows how to sell unfinished analysis as some sort of meaningful metrics that the company can't live without. But then she's gone and I'm on my own to fulfill the promises she's made.

I tried to manage the disorder with medication for seven years, but there were always uncomfortable side effects such as anxiety and nausea. Even with the pills, I was perpetually on the low side of my emotional spectrum anyway. The slightly depressed me is the form that fits most comfortably, it's my Bruce Banner, the mild-mannered scientist no one expects to turn into a raging green monster. It's what I feel is the real me and it's the one that has to do the real work, cleaning up after all the other versions of myself. And sometimes it's bad—I've created a mess like you wouldn't believe. Once, I came back from a particularly powerful high only to find I had been promoted to management. And not just one or two direct reports, but a team of fourteen individuals all expecting me to know what I was doing.

It was the end of the 1990s, and our actual manager had left for a start-up in Silicon Valley. When our weekly team meeting came around, I was there early in the conference room at the south end of the building. Yellow light broke into the room in wide slices from the burning California sun and in pointed jabs from the reflections off the waxy BMWs and Audis in the parking lot below the wall of window. But the room was always cold. The forced air from the vents tasted almost metallic.

I popped the cap off a sharp-smelling marker and pressed it to the stony surface of the whiteboard. As the room filled up, I wrote out an agenda in loopy, red letters that squeaked with each flourish. I breathed in the mercurial air of the room. The fiery light, elevating odour, and silver cold quickened my pulse and cleared my head, making my thoughts run high. First, I wanted to hear everyone's status, then I would lay out the week ahead and talk about changes to the schedule that were a result of a problem one of our partners had found with the software. I had no plan for the week ahead, why would I? But I was already inventing one by the time I sat down and asked Walter, on my right, to get us started by updating us on what he'd been working on. At the end of the meeting, I would introduce Luke, the division director who we would all be reporting to until a new manager could be found. Luke sat in the back of the room, away from the table, and watched.

Within a week after that meeting, Luke had come to my office to formally invite me to accept the position of manager. I imagine the team thought that Luke had asked me to play the leadership role for the meeting that day, or they were too perplexed to challenge me. They may have even felt reassured and relaxed that someone was handling things. If so, it would be one of the few things I did right in my brief career in management.

The promotion wasn't just the fault of the mania but also of the training I received when I was hospitalized. At the Batty Centre, I picked up a few important things that help me succeed in the corporate world without so much as a high school diploma. I learned how to detect what people want to hear and how to turn that into a promotion. Most importantly, I learned how to act normal, which isn't that hard considering most people are a little off themselves.

When confined to a mental ward with magnetic-lock doors and nurses who double as bouncers, when given shots and tests and pills and asked to give up mouthwash and shoelaces as contraband, a normal person does not react sanely. The sane thing to do would be to scream and throw things, make false threats, demand to speak to whoever's in charge, ask for a lawyer, pretend you know your rights, and beg everyone you come in contact with to help you escape. At least I think so. But normal people don't react that way until it's too late. They say, "This is absurd," as they unlace their shoes and hand the strings to the nurse in charge. Normal people ask, "When will I be able to make a phone call?" as they're led by the elbow by a man carrying leather straps, their loose shoes tripping them as they walk down the hall to the office with all the needles. Normal people simply try not to act crazy, even when the situation warrants it. Once you've learned that, it's easy to put up with whatever inane tasks you are called on to do at work.

When I was first admitted to the Batty Centre for bipolar disorder, I was assigned a security level of One. I had access to my room and, during the appropriate hours, the middle hall, where I attended my state-mandated classes, and the cafeteria. Every time I tried to escape, my security level would drop to Zero and I would be assigned to SAR, which meant I had to sit at a desk opposite the nurses' station from seven in the morning until nine at night. I don't know what the acronym actually stood for, but the other patients called it Sit And Rot. Eventually I would get back up to a One by not mouthing off to the nurses and by sitting quietly for a full day. Then I would sneak out of the classroom and investigate the magnetic-lock doors again until I was back on Sit And Rot.

The highest security level a patient could achieve was a Five, which allowed them to leave the premises when accompanied by another level Five. There wasn't anywhere to go within walking distance of the hospital except the market up the street, which sold pints of ice cream. But when you are on Sit And Rot and the only meal you get is swirly bread with ham and cheese twice a day, ice cream is a pretty tempting goal.

I'd meet regularly with my psychiatrist, Dr. Jennings. At first, I asked for help by telling Dr. Jennings where he could stick his chalky pills. Then I started just blatantly asking.

"What do you want me to say?" I sat on the little couch across from Dr. Jennings's desk and wrapped a loose string from the hem of my T-shirt around my finger and watched my skin turn white from the pressure.

Dr. Jennings pushed his glasses up his pulpy, mottled nose until they encroached on the undergrowth of his greying eyebrows. He scratched a few lines of text onto his pad. "We're all just here to help you, Addy. I need to know how you're doing with this medication. Is the medication making you feel different in any way?"

"I don't know. Just tell me what you want me to say. I just want to get out of here."

"Do you want to go home?" Dr. Jennings always wore a jacket and tie. He was the only person I had ever had reason to talk to who dressed like that.

"Can I?"

"You can once we've determined that you are capable of making good decisions."

"How are you going to determine that? I'm not even allowed to make any decisions in this place." I tried to read his notes, but even close up and with the right orientation, they would have been hard to make out. "Ask me a question, I'll make a decision right now. Any question."

Even if I had known what Dr. Jennings wanted me to say to show that I was normal, he would not have discharged me that day or even increased my security clearance. To get a promotion, I had to demonstrate consistently that I was already performing at the next level. It's not like a graduation where you complete a task and are rewarded with advancement. Completing a task only lets you start to prepare for a promotion. It works the same way in business.

I eventually did learn what Dr. Jennings wanted me to say, and I said it enough that I was released from the Batty Centre. He wanted to hear me talk as if I was committed to myself and to getting better. And although I wasn't then, I eventually learned why he was looking for that and why it was important.

I finally learned the importance of committing to myself years later from the corporation that promoted me to management while I was hypomanic. By the time the hypomania wore off, I had gone from being the new girl to being the new manager of a team of fourteen engineers, some of whom were old enough to be my father. I was twenty-four, a high school dropout, and completely unprepared to manage anything. When it came time to evaluate the performance of my direct reports, I wrote out what I could about what I knew of their work. Most of it was positive—but one employee, Matt, had stopped showing up for work regularly and had been garnering some complaints from other people at the company.

Shortly after reviews were over, Human Resources called me in for some questions. Matt had filed a formal complaint against me. The HR representative was a young man with stiff hair and carefully trimmed sideburns. His name was Richard and he told me to call him Ricky, which I did when I had to, but he didn't look like a Ricky to me. He certainly didn't act like a Ricky. So in my head I just called him HR. He asked me to sit. Then he leaned back in his tall leather chair and crossed one foot over a knee. His shoes were shiny and unscuffed and his socks were dark with little purple diamonds.

"If you had a problem with an employee's performance, why didn't you talk with him and develop a performance plan?" HR asked. He had a law degree from an Ivy League school on the wall behind his head. On his desk was a paper cube with orange and white sides. On each side was printed a word like "leadership" and four bullet points itemizing symptoms of that word. Bullet: influencing business. Bullet: motivating others. Bullet: decision-making. Bullet: role-modelling.

"I didn't have time?" I leaned to my left to try to read the text on the far side of the cube.

"How is an employee supposed to know if they aren't performing up to expectations if you don't communicate that to them?" HR asked. He was wearing a tie with purple stripes that matched the diamonds on his socks. I was wearing jeans and an Atari T-shirt.

"I said what the problem was in his review," I said. "I gave details. Which is what my boss said to do."

"The review shouldn't be a surprise to any of your employees."

"I don't see how it could have been a surprise." I slumped back in my plastic guest chair and stared right at him. I wanted him to fire me so that I could go home and cry and sleep and hide in my room and try to pretend none of this was happening.

"Do you think your personal feelings influenced the review you gave Matt?" HR asked.

"What do you mean? About Matt? Or just in general?"

Ricky put his hands down and looked at me with one well-waxed eyebrow raised. "About Matt."

"No, then."

HR had to determine if there were some unjust practices going on as Matt had claimed. Whether I had tried to punish Matt out of retaliation or discriminated against him for some belief he held or whether I had some prejudice against his race or age or sex. The fact that I was just a bad manager, alternating between quiet periods of avoiding people and chaotic fits of essentially "playing house" with my job, wasn't really a legal offence. It was a long investigation.

Each day that I met with HR, I had to work even later to complete my projects, answer my email, and attend to all the little things the Hulk had signed me up for. I needed to sleep, I needed to stay away from people because they exhausted me, and I needed HR to stop hassling me. Because of the problem with Matt's review and the legal actions he was threatening to take, my own review was modified from the stellar score the Hulk had elicited to a much more modest one. I started getting migraines on a near daily basis.

My job experience looked good on paper, but it didn't translate well into real life. All of the brilliance and grandeur that had propelled me up the ladder was a mirage, and when it faded, nothing had changed for the regular me. I wasn't performing at the next level, I just looked like I was. The skills I learned in the hospital were just highly specialized forms of mimicry. The Hulk is nothing more than a big green, heavily caffeinated parrot. I quit my job at the company before the next annual review cycle and enrolled at a university, an institution to which I committed myself to take full advantage.

Five years later at my new job, the one I got with my updated resumé that includes a section on education, I have my own office. I sit at my desk all day, and when people come to see me, I try to look at them even when things blink on my computer screen. When I return from my weekly one on one with my manager, Mark, I push my keyboard aside and look at the list I've made in my spiral-bound notebook. I draw little arrows next to each of the tasks on my list to reprioritize them as high or low importance. The static of randomization makes it hard to assess them. I scribble away half of the margin, blacking out double-headed arrows and question marks. I'm just buying time until the hypomania sets in, but I can't rely on the Hulk and her ramshackle approach to manufacturing a life. I'm getting better at slowing her down so that I don't get so overwhelmed, and I'm getting better at building supports along the way so that not everything comes tumbling down all at once when the hypomania leaves in the middle of a job. My Plan B is to commit to myself and my responsibilities and to try to do the best job I can with whatever qualities I possess at the time. But for now I'm still hoping that hypomania will set in before the deadline.

Code Three

SCOTT WHYTE

It was a chilly Valentine's Day in 1986 when my unmarked police car got clobbered by a Dodge pickup in a head-on highway collision. I'll never forget the lightning-fast crack and the thundering "POW!" Our car convulsed wildly in a whiteout of snow, and, conversely, loose objects within the car seemed to float in slow motion around me. I looked over at my partner, who was in the driver's seat. Shards of crumpled metal and jagged moulding surrounded him, and his eyes were frozen wide open. I didn't sense he was dead, but I knew I was alone for the rest of this ride. The windshield was gone, and we were alternatively blasted with cold air coming in or struggling to breathe as the cold air was being sucked out. We kept spinning counter-clockwise, and all I could do was fold my hands in my lap and hope for a safe stop. Our movement was finally arrested by a snowbank. The car was on fire, but at least we were safe.

I left that accident scene in an ambulance, with whiplash that plagues me to this day. I was sidelined in bed for six weeks before I could get back to work; work had been my priority back then. I carried away something else from the carnage as well. I didn't recognize it because, like whiplash, it was also invisible. The seed for post-traumatic stress disorder had been planted in me and was taking root.

I found myself in some unfamiliar trouble. I couldn't sleep. I wasn't able to turn off my thoughts. I would think something through to its end only to urgently need to start from the beginning once more. This pattern got faster and faster until it felt like being caught in a vortex over a draining sink. I was being sucked into the unknown. I called the police psychologist, told him about the accident, the workload that greeted me upon my return to the office, my newfound discomfort riding as the passenger in any police car, and my runaway thought patterns. He told me over the telephone that I was overworked and needed to take a few days off. He sent me a cassette tape with a relaxation exercise on it. I had to listen to this tape twice a day for two weeks and I would be fixed right up. A month later, I requested a transfer onto the local highway patrol unit. I needed simpler work.

I started experiencing subtle shifts in my perception. One began as a pleasant little tingle. I had been dispatched to a single vehicle accident at about 10:00 PM one winter's night. A pickup truck had wandered off the right-hand side of the road, careened into the ditch, hit a rock, and overturned. The driver, still belted in, hung upside down, clinging to life in the bitter cold. I was coming Code 3—lights, siren, and hyper-vigilant; dodging bewildered drivers, semi-trailer trucks, cows, moose, and deer. It took me an hour to get there.

I arrived to a small group of sombre attendants who were huddled together for comfort and warmth. I got out of my car and pushed through the snow as I clambered down into the ditch. I dug down with my mitts to where the window should have been. The truck was on its roof, the cab compressed and the glass broken. I looked in on the young lady. She was dead. I just happened to be on my knees when I straightened up to lean against the side of the truck. I looked up and I offered a private word, "Keep an eye open for this poor soul and welcome her when she gets there." At the very instant the message left me, a tingle began at the base of my spine. It grew in intensity as it rose slowly up my back until it finally radiated around my neck like a nice, warm scarf. It lingered for a wonderful moment before being channelled to the base of my skull. I was stunned in the wake of its ecstasy. What was it? Was it normal? I hoped so! But what a dangerous bit of denial this turned out to be. It laid the groundwork for the next ten years of my declining health.

I was by no means silent for those ten years. I called out for help along the way, but the system failed to recognize what was happening to me. I had bouts of insecurity and fear, occasional nightmares, and felt, at times, like I was having heart attacks. I went into the hospital to get checked out and I was always dismissed with the same advice: *come back when we can witness your complaint in action.* The blasted attacks always happened away from the hospital. On the way to some police call-outs I shook uncontrollably behind the wheel. I felt the anticipation of going into something unknown, possibly hazardous, but it wasn't fear I was feeling. I felt cold and was shivering in July and August. I reported these issues to the doctors, but they shrugged their shoulders and didn't offer any insights into my symptoms—their advice was to come back when I was actually shivering.

I moved from 100 Mile House to Prince Rupert, British Columbia. I was placed in a regional serious crime unit of only four people with a huge area to cover. At the same time, the Royal Canadian Mounted Police (RCMP) in British Columbia had been going through some painful structural and financial issues. The "in-house" squabbles and the stress being created by those little turf wars were beyond anything I had ever witnessed out on the street. We were a busy unit trying to operate in a toxic environment and not everybody in the sandbox was playing well together.

My boss (who didn't like me) got suspended and banned from the office pending an internal investigation. The second in-charge (I liked him) got transferred to another location and was replaced with an idiot. The third officer was promoted and moved to a new posting without being replaced. Eventually the idiot was also transferred without being replaced and that finally left me to fend for myself.

I managed to survive for a while, but ultimately I was pulled under by depression and the constant gloom of the third wettest climatic zone on Earth. The police psychologist, over a cup of coffee this time, told me I was in need of a little boost and advised me to get a prescription for Prozac from my family doctor. My doctor opted instead to do some tests; he discovered my thyroid gland was having problems and we worked on fixing that rather than feeding me Prozac. After a while, though, my world continued closing in on me, the pressures were everywhere; it took everything I had to move in slow motion.

Something new and unexpected happened as I was plodding through two large, historical case files. One was a confirmed murder. The second will probably always rank as a missing person status until somebody finds some physical evidence of foul play, but hey—after ten years of hearing nothing from a thirteen-year-old girl who was last seen hitchhiking home along a notorious stretch of Highway 16 (the Highway of Tears)—I'd say her disappearance was the result of a murder too.

I had been asked to clear a "person of interest" (let's call him Fred) from the confirmed murder case, to better isolate another identified suspect. This was something we did routinely, but Fred began to connect with the victim in ways that outshone the favoured suspect. I found new energy, dedicated more hours, lost track of my sleep, and sure enough, I began connecting Fred to more than just one victim. I saw connections forming to murders that other units were investigating too. This was exciting! The evidence was unfolding right before my eyes! I had tripped onto the one-stop-shop solution for many of the unsolved murders throughout British Columbia and western Canada.

I found a rural property that had, at one time, been occupied by

Fred and another guy who is now dead. I had learned that Fred and his buddy had been bragging about an infatuation for the missing girl, and Fred let it slip to one too many people that he'd taken part in killing someone. This piece of property also matched the same description being provided by no fewer than three psychics. These psychics then told me where to look for the missing girl. My job as the investigator was to dig.

I frantically dug several holes to find that girl's remains. One of the psychics sat beside me while I was digging the last hole. She was suddenly in conversation with the ghost of the girl I was searching for. The missing girl had a message for me. Her ghost was grateful and said I had successfully identified one of her killers, but there wasn't any evidence in the ground I was disturbing. This was a huge letdown; I had been probing for weeks! The ghost also said that we needed to leave the hillside or we would be contending with a "dead guy's ghost"—he was apparently pure evil and not at all happy about the number of divots being left all over his hill.

That night, like the two or three nights before it, I wasn't able to sleep. My thoughts were spinning wildly. I was scared spit-less over what I was experiencing and nothing made any sense.

In the morning, I went into the local police office, sat in a chair, and just stared at the wall. I was trying to make sense of what was happening when it dawned on me. The psychic's name was the keystone! I was dizzy and craved fresh air. I felt an internal shifting of perception that scared me. Suddenly I realized my destiny was to be intertwined with the second coming of Jesus Christ. I inwardly screamed that this couldn't be right. I panicked. Something was definitely wrong. I felt the urgent need to drive into Prince George. It would be a six-hour drive from where I was in Smithers, but the closest help was there and nowhere else. I needed a preacher or a shrink.

During that lonely drive my thoughts were merciless. I had a number of involved conversations with God. I didn't actually hear his voice, but I could ask him "yes or no" questions and I got responses to each one. Those delicious rivers of tingling energy that had been innocently running up and down my spine for years were now addictively available for the asking. "Hey, God, does this mean what I think it does?" A current of pleasure flowing from the bottom meant "Yes" and "No" came down from the top. Both strokes were exquisite and I just loved the ebb and flow of this energy.

I was so preoccupied with my thoughts and ballooning flight of fantasy that I wandered into the path of an oncoming logging truck and then later a B-train transport. I was convinced I was on a mission from God. I had been chosen to find, fight, and eliminate evil. It did not escape me that I was armed with a semi-automatic weapon, worked in plain clothes, and drove a "ghost car." While I had the direct line to my new boss, I still wanted a second opinion before committing myself to further action. That's what caused me to veer twice back into my own lane. I wasn't ready for suicide yet.

My second opinion arrived through the teamwork of a psychologist and a psychiatrist of my own choosing in Prince George. Their diagnosis was bipolar mood disorder type II, a serious mental illness. I was sick and stuck without psychiatric services on the edge of the continent, in an isolated posting called Prince Rupert. This port city had no direct flight service to Prince George, and ten hours of challenging highway lay between the two locations. I had to drive that distance every time I needed to see my doctors. The most obvious solution was to grant me a compassionate medical transfer, but the RCMP flatly refused, citing lack of money.

On the date of my departure from duty, I was just one day shy of realizing my first promotion, which would have meant a transfer closer to help. I had passed all the prerequisites and held a solid footing; I'd scored forty-second in a ranking of fourteen hundred hopefuls. I had earned this step-up well before hitting my breaking point. It would have meant a bump in pay and an increase to my eventual pension too, but it was all to be placed out of my reach. Once I realized the promotion was going to be denied, I then sought any form of compromise to negotiate the earliest possible transfer from an isolated posting to a place where I could be closer to my professional caregivers. I was flatly refused time and time again by one stubborn, faceless administrator—an officer in our headquarters—who was playing "hard ball with a cripple." No money, no mercy. The only way I could get closer to the kind of help I required was to request a "voluntary" medical discharge. It didn't feel voluntary and it lacked the compassion I had come to expect from this world-renowned organization.

My divorce from the force took place after twenty-three years of long and decorated service. It was not how I had envisioned my retirement. The people I had worked with for years fell silent around me. I tried to reconnect only to find the conversations strained, shallow, and short. These social fractures were perhaps some of the most painful realities of my existence. For those sitting on the sidelines watching a co-worker, friend, or acquaintance falling into the hole of a mental illness, a caring call or even a card might resolve some of the isolation created by the stigma of this illness.

My first challenge was to stabilize with medications, which wasn't a precision operation. The psychiatrist prescribed a pill and then sat back to see what happened. The first six guesses using Paxil, Effexor, Nardil, Levoprome, to name the few I can remember, found me retching, or writhing in a fetal ball surrounded by an anxiety so crushing I could scarcely move, or blasting off into new heights of manic explosion. I am very fortunate—pill number seven was Depakote (Epival) and it worked for me. Seven attempts at finding the right medication is a comparatively low number, I've been told. I can now live with the side effects, and the benefits have been well worth the risks.

There is a solid system of disability pension for those physically hurt in the line of duty; the same cannot be said for those who psychologically suffer. My claim for whiplash was accepted immediately, without question. At the same time, I was summarily rejected on the issue of my mental illness. I had to appeal that decision within a formalized timeline, hire a lawyer, and go through the added stress of appearing before a tribunal. I had *to prove* that I was in fact mentally ill and that my illness was duty-related. I openly wept before that tribunal at the additional strain it had placed upon me. I won a partial pension in the end but at an aggravated and personal cost.

Then came the insurance fights. There had been no choice other than to pay into the force's long-term disability insurance plan. I did so with a blind faith. It turned out that long-term translated into just two years. The coverage also limited my total income from all sources to 70 per cent of what I had been earning. Dealing with the insurance company was nothing short of cruel, particularly when my illness was exacerbated by stress. I was left to wander for two years in a haze of low self-esteem, restricted income, and confusion. It socially isolated me from everyone I had known. Everything required an argument and I was sick of it. It was all a catalyst for more depression.

There was no map to show me the way so I made up my own. I decided to give college a try. I was attacked on the very first day with new anxieties. I couldn't handle the crowds. I felt as though everybody could see right through me. I couldn't hide that I was a *sicko* and different from the *norm*. I couldn't handle a full course load. I had to scale back. I felt weak, worthless, and nothing came easily anymore.

It was actually a few words of sombre advice that got me started in the right direction. Dr. Grimmer, the psychologist I had found in Prince George, said, "Scott, if you want to *survive*, you need to learn a few things about stress and how to deal with it." She saw that I had a trunk full of stressors and not one positive way to handle any of it. I needed nothing short of a lifestyle makeover. My first steps were to explore my feelings, learn my triggers, and get to a state of being proactive rather than reactive. I discovered a direct relationship between stress and the symptoms of my mental illness. My illness got worse when my stressors stacked up and my illness retreated when my stressors were mitigated. My medications were only a fraction of the treatment needed to regain and sustain my health. The bigger picture incorporated problem-solving, regular exercise, deep relaxation, smarter nutrition, a new social support network, and a healthy amount of sleep. Controlling my stress through these means has given me a measurable degree of control over my own illness.

I enrolled into a program hosted by the BC Schizophrenia Society called Bridges. It was a brilliant concept of peer-to-peer training that got my recovery going in some very positive directions. I found community support and got active. My healthier mission became one of reducing the social stigma that hangs over this illness.

I spoke on the local radio station many times and was featured in a number of newspaper articles. I provided education to the community about mental illness through my new employment with the Canadian Mental Health Association. The people I came to know through this organization helped me to get over more hurdles than I can count.

I know now that I can no longer ride through life using Code 3 responses. Blaring my lights and blasting the siren is just too stressful. Instead I gain balance, strength, and structure from my work. I train peace and probation officers to better understand mental illness and consider using more effective crisis intervention techniques. I lead a small group of brave people who share in a "lived experience of a mental illness." Our panel speaks to the officers in an outreach effort to provide a better understanding of our illness to those who tend to meet us only in our times of crisis. I also teach a stress-management component in which officers can better understand the role stress is playing within the crises they must attend to and show them that they, too, are vulnerable to the grasp of a mental illness—by virtue of the Code 3 environment they work in. The result has been to establish a newfound empathy and a better understanding for everyone I instruct.

I have a renewed sense of purpose, belonging, and comfort. Recovery from a mental illness is a series of "baby steps." The little victories, acquired with every step, add up to something worthwhile.

Crazy

One Woman's Search for Sanity

GAIL MARLENE SCHWARTZ

(Upstage left there is an easel with a white tablet and the word CRAZY *written on it. There is also a wooden folding chair centre stage and a* TV *monitor with a* DVD *player set up stage right. There is a small props table with a bunny, a paintbrush, cards, and a prayer book. At the top of the show, before curtain, GAIL is mingling with the audience, finishing preparations. An announcement is made, then VOLUNTEER pushes play on the video, showing the conductor sequence. GAIL enters, riding a child's bicycle. She parks upstage centre/right and turns to the audience.)*

GAIL:

When I was five, I spent fifty minutes each week with the first of my eighteen therapists, Dr. Aaron Abramson. My parents explained that they were sending me to Dr. A because I was being a bad girl and Dr. A would help me be a good girl. They said he would teach me how to express my feelings. (*She crosses to easel.*) My mother would tell me it was time for my Wednesday afternoon appointment . . .

(GAIL *transforms into her five-year-old self and shrieks, clinging to the easel.*)

"Noooooooooooooooooooooooooooooooo!!!!!!!!!!!!!!"

(*She rises, adult.*) Express my feelings . . . APPROPRIATELY. When we finally got to the office, she hauled me in and dropped me into Dr. A's beanbag chair. The doctor had a kind bearded face that I didn't want to spend fifty minutes staring at. The first thing I always did was get up, take the easel that stood in the corner, and plunk it down between his chair and mine. (*She takes the easel and moves it slightly downstage.*) He would say to me,

(*as Dr. A*)

Gail, would you like to talk about how you feel about that easel?

(GAIL *moves behind the easel and slowly gives the finger over the top. She moves out to the props table to talk to the audience.*)

But he never stopped trying.

(*She picks up the BUNNY and goes back to the easel.*)

"Gail, Mr. Bunny is feeling happy to see you. He wants to know how you're feeling today."

(GAIL *goes behind the easel, drops a second bunny, with a noose around its neck, over the top. She walks back in front.*)

He seemed to have an endless supply of creative tactics designed to get me to open up. (*She goes to the props table and trades the bunnies for the paintbrush.*)

"Gail, how would you like to do a special art project? It's called, 'How I'm Feeling.'"

(GAIL *goes in back of the easel and wipes the brush loudly against the pad, simulating painting. She slowly shows, above the top of the pad, a colourful picture of a pig with Hitler's face cut out and superimposed on*

the face of the pig; in childlike lettering at the bottom, it reads, "Dr. A."
She emerges from behind the easel and goes to the props table.)

I couldn't believe it—he never yelled at me and he never gave up. (*She trades the paintbrush for the cards.*) Finally, after weeks of failed attempts . . .

"Gail, today we're going to write feeling cards. If you write one to me, I'll write you back."

(She moves behind the easel and writes. She slowly walks out, looking at the card and then at the audience, showing the card, which reads, "MAD.")

He was the first person I told. Suddenly, the Big Bad Wolf became my trusted confidante. We wrote notes and passed them back and forth across the easel. One time, I even invited him to sit with me on my side and help me paint a picture: a self-portrait.

(She suddenly notices, out loud, how dirty the floor is. She goes and gets the broom from the props table. She sweeps. She improvises out loud about needing to make sure the stage is clean, etc. At one point she stops.)

Crazy scares me.

(She sees that the bike is dirty and crosses to clean it with her hanky.)

My Aunt Stephanie was a doctor, on the other side of crazy—the white coat wearing, patient seeing, prescription writing side. She thought I had a chemical imbalance. Aunt Stephanie loved my creative side and wanted to see me succeed; she was convinced this was the way. So she sent me to see her psychiatrist friend, therapist number fourteen, Dr. Isaac Finkelstein. I couldn't believe it, a Jewish shrink, out there in the shticks of Vermont. His steady voice reminded me of afternoons with Grandpa Sid on his front porch in Westbury, playing twenty questions when I was nine.

After we chatted about New York for a few minutes, the doctor asked me about my symptoms:

(as Dr. Finkelstein)

Is your sleep irregular?

Do you feel nauseous?

Are you irritable during the day?

Do you have suicidal thoughts and feelings?

Do you worry and obsess?

Do you feel helpless and hopeless?

Do you tremble and shake?

Do you have irrational fears?

(GAIL walks left to the easel and turns the page, revealing the list of questions. She checks each one off, thinking while she goes, the checking-off action becoming faster and faster.)

Yes.

Yes.

Yes.

Yes.

Yes.

Yes.

Yes.

Yes.

GENERALIZED ANXIETY DISORDER!!! It was a perfect diagnosis. *(She crosses to centre.)* After fifty minutes, he sent me home with two prescriptions and a list of five more therapists to call.

But, Doc, if it's biochemical, why do I need therapy?

I can't remember what he said.

(She goes to the easel.)

Oh, sorry, I'm kind of an organization freak . . . my favourite Sunday outing is wandering the aisles of Staples, hunting for that perfect desk caddy . . . I get so absorbed in my lists . . . sometimes I lose myself.

I was held by therapist number five, Dr. Julie Hannaford. At thirteen, the anxiety pulsing through my body got so high one day that it broke inside, like a forest fire. Evenings brought screaming matches between my parents or between my mother and me. And school, which had once been a refuge, had turned into another danger zone. Dana Williams and Eleanor Eichler, sitting behind me in math class, whispered names into my ear. "Gaaaaay . . . lezzie . . ." and the worst—"towering inferno!!!" Sometimes Eleanor would wad up little bits of paper, roll them around in her mouth, and then spit them into my short curls, where they stuck like snowflakes. Both girls would cackle in low voices, escaping the teacher's notice. My mother would get home from work and ask me what was wrong. When I told her she would say, "Just ignore them. If you let it get to you, you're asking for more." I knew I had to fix the situation, but I didn't know how.

On that day, they are teasing me like always but this time Eleanor whispers, "We're gonna get you on your way home from school—we're gonna take all your clothes and leave you on the side of the road." They sit back in their seats and crack up. This time the teacher tells them to shush but immediately gets back to his fractions. At that moment, I feel something inside of me ignite and my bones turn into sticks, crackling and popping in the flames. I get a ride home and know I have to make it stop. Cut off the air supply. The fire will sink. I can rest. I get inside the house and am alone, thank goodness, my parents at their jobs, my sister at band practice. I grab a bottle of Aspirin and Smokey the Bear's image pops into my head: only you, only you, only you . . . I imagine myself in the ground, calm, cool, quiet. I pour pills into my wobbly hand. Only you. Put them in and put it out. Only you. I imagine dark, comforting earth cuddling me like a cushion. I throw the white tablets back onto my tongue. Only you. I grab the ceramic mug with the toothpaste smudges. Only you. Drink. Only you. Twentyish tablets slide down my throat in slow motion. I imagine lying in a cool lake, floating, fireless. I sit on the toilet and wait.

Then, scene change, I am meeting with Julie for an emergency appointment. My parents, furious and hysterical, had brought me in. "Am I going to die?" She tells me I haven't taken enough to hurt myself. The realization sinks in. I start to cry. She asks me if I want to be held. I am surprised—nobody has ever asked me that before and it actually seems like a pretty good idea. She offers me her hand and I take it . . . and then she folds me into her, gently pushing my face into her blue fuzzy sweater. We sit like that for the rest of the session, taking occasional breaks to breathe.

For the first time in months the burning subsides.

(She does a movement sequence with the chair and transitions into standing.)

On my thirty-fifth birthday, in a session with therapist number sixteen, Penelope Upjohn, I decided to change my identity. I'd always been a seeker—therapy, meditation, organic food, non-violent communication. At thirty-five, I decided I didn't want to be a seeker anymore—I wanted to be a finder. I no longer cared why I broke up my last relationship by calling ten, sometimes twenty times in a half-hour, panicked that my partner was in bed with her ex. I was no longer interested in understanding my insistent urge to take a flame to the soft underside of my arm and scorch it black. I didn't want to delve into the psychological roots of my panic attacks that led to lost sleep, lost work, lost love. And I no longer wanted to explore early patterns, repressed anger, blocked energy. I just wanted an answer . . . and a solution.

So, I bought my very own copy of the DSM. The DSM is the United States' medical establishment's clinical guide to every diagnosable mental illness to date. I started reading and made a list of the mental illnesses that I thought might fit me. (*She gets a scrolled list out of her pocket. She removes the coloured paper clip and the paper unscrolls, revealing a very long list. She begins reading.*)

Attention deficit hyperactivity disorder.

Separation anxiety disorder.

Avoidant disorder of childhood.

Overanxious disorder.

Developmental arithmetic disorder.

Gender identity disorder of childhood.

Gender identity disorder of adulthood, nontranssexual type.

Identity disorder.

Stereotype habit disorder.

Organic mood syndrome.

Organic anxiety syndrome.

Organic personality syndrome.

Paranoid disorder.

Manic episode.

Major depressive episode.

Bipolar disorder mixed.

Cyclothemia.

Dysthemia.

Panic disorder.

Panic disorder with agoraphobia.

Social phobia.

Obsessive compulsive disorder.

Post-traumatic stress disorder.

Generalized anxiety disorder.

(She moves to kneeling stage right of the chair and with breath starts to tear the list.)

I remember being four years old and needing ever so desperately to learn to ride my shiny new two-wheeler bike. I would get up at 5:00 AM every day to practise. Scraped knees, bruised elbows, even a scratch on my cornea from a tree branch didn't stop me. Somehow the injuries gave me more determination. I'll never forget the day I got it. It was a Saturday morning and my dad was out practising with me. He would hold the seat and run with me for a few feet and then let me go. Usually I'd get in about five or six rotations of the pedals and then lose my balance. But then he got me up and going. I gripped those handlebars, focused, determined. The wind was blowing leaves around and I was wearing my favourite yellow flowered dress. I felt my father release me and I began pedalling as I had before. But this time, I felt myself being lifted, carried. *(She gathers the little pieces and gets up, crosses in front of the sheet.)* I had the sensation of flying I would feel in my dreams. Balance kicked in. I got it! I got it! I'm soaring!

(At the end of the monologue, she twirls around with the little torn pieces and releases them around her; they fall like snowflakes. GAIL collapses centre stage, then lifts herself up with great effort to sitting.)

It's December 2002. I am off the medication that therapist number seventeen, Lila Zorn, had prescribed, after extensive weaning. I am unemployed, in the middle of a divorce, living in a town where I know nobody. I am responsible for bills I have no idea how I will pay. My family knows of my situation, but nobody makes any offers. I know I am responsible for what happens to me and I flop around mentally about my situation. "We make our own reality." "Everything happens for a reason." "We manifest what is inside of us." I reluctantly agree to have sex with a man I meet in the mall in a loose arrangement that includes cash. That month my bills are paid.

The fire returns to my body after the affair. My apartment is covered with dirty dishes, empty Diet Pepsi cans, old newspapers with job ads clipped out, and laundry I do not have the energy to do. I lie down on the couch, where I spend most of my days. I turn on the TV and imitate my teenaged siblings, Look, Ma, I'm channel surfing. I become mesmerized in the images, the slasher movie, the international figure skating championship, the Woody Allen film. After four hours I turn the TV off, feeling loopy. I draw a bath and hear my voice free-association swearing, shouting, making percussive sounds with my lips, singing at the top of my lungs. Who is this? Have I fallen off the deep end? I sing more and laugh, playing in my bath, and then the part of me watching myself falls away. Now I'm 100 per cent crazy, rules of behaviour gone, and I pass through humming to naming each of my knuckles to being President Bush addressing the nation to saying the word *dissect* over and over and over until it is unrecognizable.

I pick up the razorblade from the side of the tub and stare at it. Then I start to cry. I cry for myself. I cry for my aunt, my grandmother, and my two great uncles. I cry for my sister. I cry for my father. And finally I cry for my mother, for the lasting vision of my mother, chasing her six-year-old down the street, angry, terrified, and alone.

Then I sleep. (*She moves to the bike and sits/leans on it.*) The next day, I get the urge to call my mother and for the first time in my life tell her I love her. I pick up the phone, start to dial, and then put down the receiver. Instead, I walk into town, noticing the candles in my neighbour's window, the stars in the sky, getting lost in the texture of the woman's hair in front of me, having trouble suppressing my smile.

(*She breathes and puts her head down, then after a pause looks up, noticing her watch.*)

(*to the audience*) Well, I'm afraid our time is just about up for today.

This is definitely my favourite part of the show—cleanup! (*She gets busy sweeping the stage.*)

Sometimes after the show somebody will ask me, "So, did you find a cure for your anxiety?" I never know what to say.

(*She suddenly stops sweeping, seeing the pile of torn-up papers in a different light. She drops the broom, scoops up the papers, and gently blows air at them, watching the little flutters with joy. Final video begins, showing a young Gail practising riding her two-wheel bike—the same bike she has onstage.*)

Hey, have you seen those new binders from Staples? They're completely transparent. If I ride fast enough, I just might make it there before closing.

(*She flips the easel to the last page, which reads, "An End" and exits.*)

BLACKOUT

Late Summer, Early Fall, as Told to the Dead of Winter

MEREDITH DARLING

January 27, 1994, and the room smells of apple blossoms, my favourite incense. I'm at the glass-topped table at the far end of my room at my mother's house in Ottawa. On the table beside the plate of cookies sits a pot of tea, a jar of honey, and my cup and saucer. I call this little nook Café Mérédith. The experts say a café is the best place to write, and I have a great imagination. My spiral notebook is open and I'm trying to write. My mind, however, drifts.

Ever since my *illness*, I've been trying to write. This means spending hours poring over books that I hope will somehow tell me what to do. I've searched through the works of everyone from Natalie Goldberg to Anthony Robbins. I search to see if Edgar Cayce has any advice for timid young writers. The books fail me, and I head down the street to the Occult Shop to see what magic and astrology can do for me. I ache for the days, not so long ago, when I believed in magic, when I had faith in astrology, when I was proud to have my moon in Pisces. Lunar Pisceans are poets, psychics, and healers.

I long especially for some kind of spell that will teach me how to write masterpiece screenplays so I can get into film school. But I find none.

The previous summer I believed I had mastered the universe. Actually what had happened was slightly less glamorous: I had *cracked*.

■   ■   ■

My story begins three years before, at a time when I was eighteen years old and first meeting Sunshine Jones. Sunshine was passing through Ottawa on her summer travels and was staying with my friend Rain. We met in the alley where the punks hung out at the ByWard Market. She was the child of hippies, and said she'd been on her own since she was twelve. She looked too cosmopolitan for Ottawa in her black catsuit, army boots, curly blond hair, and big green eyes. She thought I was cool with my Morticia Addams hair and Metallica T-shirt.

A few days after our meeting, I phoned Rain and Sunshine answered. I was in tears before I got my story out, upset my application to film school had been turned down. Sunshine suggested we hitchhike to Montreal together. I'd been trying to make it to Montreal for more than a year, not easy with my mother standing in the way. So I packed my bag, met Sunshine behind the Rideau Centre, and we headed out.

"I can stay with my brother," I lied, knowing Donnie wouldn't put up with me for long.

When we got to Montreal, Sunshine invited me to her place. It was like a real home, not like some student's place. And her boyfriend, Paul, with the massive dreadlock that hung from the back of his head like a baguette, was impressive. Though he was not impressed with me.

"She's not staying here, is she?" he asked Sunshine while I sat in the living room.

Ignoring Paul's protest, we agreed that I would stay at their St. Viateur Street apartment until the lease ran out at the end of the month. She confided to me that she was getting bored with Paul and had started seeing a drummer named Jacques. "Let's get a new apartment together," she said. "That'll make it easier to break it off with Paul."

It was too late for me to register as a full-time student at Concordia, and I was upset at not being able to get into Film Production. I cried to Sunshine, "I've never not been in school." My whole sense of self-worth was based on being in school. This was hard for Sunshine to understand. She'd gone to high school for two weeks and quit. But somehow when she came to Montreal, she'd talked her way into the hippie-flavoured New School at Dawson.

■ ■ ■

Soon after we moved in together I learned that Sunshine believed her shit literally did not stink. This she claimed was because she ate plenty of curry.

According to her, the reason I had to wear glasses and she didn't was that she got enough vitamin A. I'd taken grade thirteen biology, and now I was taking this from a girl who spelled *believe* b-e-l-e-a-v-e.

Sunshine thought the world revolved around her.

I could not get the apartment clean enough for her. She described me to her friends as a lurker and a drooler. And after I'd said, "They call St. Lawrence Street *the main* because it used to be the main street of the Jewish community," I was somehow racist.

The last straw came at Halloween. I was all set to wear my new high-gloss boots for the first time. They had cost me two hundred dollars and went all the way up to my hips. Sunshine had wanted to borrow them for a party and I had said no, I would be wearing them that night. I had a feeling she would take them, so I left a note for her that morning: "Sunshine—DO NOT take my boots!!!"

She took them anyway. I called the police and reported them stolen. "It's a civil matter," they told me. "You'll have to take care of it yourself." She returned the boots the next day and the heel was coming off one of them. When Sunshine finally left, she took with her what she wanted (whether or not it actually belonged to her), and she left the rest of the junk behind for me to clean up. "Oh well," I said to myself, "I'll never have to think about Sunshine Jones again."

■ ■ ■

Two years later on a Sunday in August, I learned the news about Sunshine.

I had received yet another rejection letter from Concordia film school, but I'd put down a backup choice, English, and had been accepted. Still, I was not happy and longed to have some sort of glimpse of my future. One thing that seemed to be working was the self-improvement campaign I'd embarked on, even though self-help books were not in my budget. I was completely broke and hoped a little fasting would clear the mind.

So I was literally starving as I headed to Mount Royal to listen to the Tam-Tams—the spontaneous drumming circle that gathers most Sundays. That's when I saw her. She was just up the street, heading toward me. I hadn't seen her in two years, but I had heard about her show on the college radio station. The day was too bright for ill feelings. I figured it was time to let bygones be bygones and when we met, I hugged her.

"Hey," I said. "What have you been up to? I've missed you."

She tossed her naturally curly blond hair. "I went to Europe last summer, and then last spring I was in Toronto. My mother directed a film for the NFB and I was in it."

"What film?" I asked, my curiosity piqued.

"It's called *The Sunshine Girl*. That's who I played, the sunshine girl." She beamed.

"That's great," I said, almost not lying. "You know I got into Concordia—English."

"So did I—Film Production."

"Oh really? How?" I struggled to keep my cool.

"A fluke, I guess," she said.

We toured around the mountain with her new boyfriend, my stomach growling the whole time. Then I went back to my cramped little one-room apartment above a Mexican restaurant. The implications of Sunshine's news had not yet sunk in.

■ ■ ■

Problems began a week later, when I started to try to piece together the puzzle of life by drawing up astrological charts. Sunshine's sun was in Aries and her moon was in Cancer; her signs ruled in both the sun and the moon—no wonder she was so lucky. I was anxious to find out what my family could do to help themselves, to find out why we never seemed to have any of the good fortune that Sunshine and her family did.

I don't know how many days and nights I sat in the middle of my tiny apartment with a mess of books strewn around me. I had everything from an old copy of *Everything You've Always Wanted to Know About Energy But Were Too Weak to Ask*, by 1970s guru Naura Hayden, to the complete works of Deepak Chopra, to Shirley MacLaine's *Out on a Limb*. I had practically bought out the entire occult, health, and psychology sections of the downtown Coles and proceeded to read them all—all at once.

At a certain point I began to feel euphoric. I believed that I was *seeing things for the first time*. This I decided was because I had achieved *Personal Transformation*. I wondered if this feeling was happening to people all over the planet. It must be the New Age, I reasoned excitedly—of course, this is the dawning of the Age of Aquarius! This weird feeling is *self-realization*.

I made an attempt to document my madness. I scribbled down my thoughts like a maniac on the backs of essays, photocopied screenplays, whatever I could find. When I ran out of paper, I began to write on whatever surface I could find, walls and floor included. The books said to listen to that little voice inside me, my intuition. Now that I had begun to listen, I could hear these voices. I figured that they must be my *spirit guides* and they were giving me important information—I was psychic after all! I was channelling *universal truths*. I wrote them down, one after the other, on note cards. "I do not need food," I wrote. "I do not need sleep."

It was near midnight when I came to the realization that I was a witch. The word *energy* took on an entirely new meaning and I began to believe that I had special powers.

The ideas that I was trying to preserve came more and more quickly, and I scribbled frantically to get them all down. GUIDES PLEASE SLOW DOWN, I wrote on the wall, believing that these *entities* would be able to see my message.

In the middle of the night, *The Plan* was uncovered. I saw that at the heart of every great cultural phenomenon there was at least one suspicious-looking girl. These girls were witches. I believed I could *sniff out the trend* and I was the witch at the centre. The time had come for The Montreal Phenomenon—all the bands, French and English, would get together and form the Montreal Sound. My brother Donnie would be their leader; the artist behind the style— he would finally get some recognition. We would all be famous! It would start with my friends from the Concordia Communications Department coming with their cameras to document the bands playing while my brother painted and directed them. I had to get ready. I covered my face with white zit cream; the photographers would be coming soon. This is how fame happens! I had finally figured it out! It happens through The Power of Positive Thinking and it happens literally overnight.

It was at this point that I began to get extremely paranoid. I looked around the room and discovered that the *Energy* book was missing, along with my *ABC of Witchcraft*. Things were getting *zapped up*. I began to believe that the other witches could tune into my thoughts and discover my secrets. I had to act fast.

I burst out the door and ran all the way to Donnie's place.

Shaking Donnie awake, I tried to explain to him what was happening and what his role was.

"Isn't that a bit unrealistic, Meredith," he said, yawning. "I think you're a bit confused. Who's giving you this information?"

"The promoters," I said, realizing that he would not understand the concept of guides. "I know the promoters."

"Come on, I don't believe you." He squinted in the darkness. "And what's with that white paint all over your face?"

"Donnie, my boy!" The words tumbled out of my mouth in a voice I did not believe was my own. "You Virgos have no faith. Don't you know who I am? Donnie, my boy, it's your great Grandpa Lashmar come back from the grave to tell you that you are going to be a great artist!"

Donnie groaned and rolled his eyes back into his head. "Why does my family have to be such a pack of lunatics?" He looked at me. "You're insane, babe. Insane."

Donnie took me back to my apartment and called my mother to come from Ottawa to get me. I showed him my *universal truths*.

"These are *catch phrases*," he said.

"But things are getting zapped up," I told him.

"Meredith, anything could get zapped up in here, this place is a mess!"

Donnie produced a horse pill, which I took and finally dozed off. When I awoke to bright sunlight, my mother had arrived.

■ ■ ■

It was back in Ottawa that I came to believe I was the *Second Coming*. We had gone straight to the holistic doctor. I told her all about my problem; that I had got *The Cosmic Joke* and had discovered I was a witch.

"Well, then," said the doctor, "you must know all about auras."

"Yes I do," I replied, thrilled that she could relate to me.

"Then you must know that you have a very sensitive aura and you must protect it."

"I understand," I said. She must have checked my chart, I thought. She must know I'm sensitive because my moon is in Pisces. "But I was going to make films," I said.

"You will be able to make films. You must take the time now to strengthen yourself," said the doctor.

"But I was going to Concordia in the fall. I have to switch my courses. I have to take a film course in the Communications Department that's taught by the Jesuit priest who's a judge at the Cannes and Venice film festivals."

"I know exactly what to do," the doctor said, picking up the phone. "You can go back out to your mother in the waiting room. I'll call the school and everything will be taken care of." She gave us a prescription for niacin that my mother filled at the drugstore on the way home.

By that evening, back in my room, I figured it out. The doctor was phoning the Jesuit priest because she knew him. She was a Jesuit in disguise and had been waiting for me. There was a network of people ready to get the ball rolling for *The Big Picture*. Sunshine had been accepted into Film because she knew me. The Film and Communications Departments at Concordia University were going to play a joke on the planet to give the world back its faith. I was to play the role of Jesus for the media. I saw myself on *Oprah* and saw Donnie painting me.

Then I saw something I didn't like. I saw Sunshine Jones getting an Academy Award for the movie she made about me.

In my pyjamas, I tore out of the house and into the street. I had to get the message out to that Jesuit professor that I would not be part of *The Picture* if Sunshine Jones was in it. I ran around the corner but then froze in my tracks. The Jesuit was controlling my every move. I was like a puppet on a string, a puppet of the universe.

My mother's car pulled up.

"Tell the Jesuits," I shouted, "it's a fluke that Sunshine Jones is in *The Picture*. I quit if she doesn't get out!" I was the one who had mastered the laws of metaphysics; without me there would be no Picture.

"Get in the car, dear," my mother said. "We can get the Jesuits' number from the hospital."

At Psychiatric Emergency, the doctor did not believe that I had secret information concerning a conspiracy against the world going on at Concordia University. She did not understand that I was *The 20th Century Joke.*

"You can come in of your own free will or we will have to commit you," said the doctor.

"Fine then, commit me! That's a good one!" I pictured myself on *Oprah.* I wore a wig and sunglasses and on the screen beneath my image was the caption, "Woman who believes she is Jesus Christ."

"How did you come to get this job?" asks Oprah.

"Well, Oprah," I say, "I had to be committed."

■   ■   ■

"You are optimistic, idealistic, and dramatic, and when things get boring, you like to stir them up." That's what the psychological tests they gave me at the hospital had to say; but they didn't give the results to me until I was almost recovered.

I spent nearly three months in the hospital.

The doctors tried God-knows-how-many antipsychotic medications before I made it into the fifth-floor experimental ward, where I tested the new atypical drug risperidone that brought me back to reality.

■   ■   ■

January 27, 1994, and the phone rings at Café Mérédith. I let it ring. I know it's Sunshine; I left a message on her answering machine for her to call me collect. Word gets around; I have some damage control to do.

Sane now, I can separate dreams from reality. I am still entranced, though, by the notion of being able to see the future. I toy with the idea as I sit here. Beneath my window, the pawprints of some unknown wild creatures have marked a giant X in the snow.

Can one see the future? You know, they say Lunar Pisces are psychic.

Life with My Mongrel

LYNNE VAN LUVEN

Her face crumples before I have time to close my office door, her hands fly up to cover her eyes, her thin shoulders start to heave. I usher her to a chair by the window, push the pink box of Scotties tissue closer, sit down across from her. By now she's sobbing: huge, juddering gasps that erupt from deep inside, the kind she's likely been holding back for weeks, the kind she probably thinks will never stop now that she's broken down and let them out. I watch, suspecting what's to come.

It's mid-March: Meltdown Month. I've been a university professor for almost three decades, long enough to recognize signs of student stress: absence from classes, semi-dopey presence in class, missing assignments, sketchy answers, forgotten appointments, shoddy drafts of articles. Sometimes, students muddle through. Other times, they fall apart, sink into confusion, simply stop coping. Sometimes, I can see a crash coming and intervene in time. Other times, distracted by my own life, I don't catch on soon enough. Sometimes I feel frustrated: since professors are not surrogate parents, I can't intrude beyond the semi-official connection of classroom-related discussions and assignments. Over the years,

I've had to teach myself an appropriate protocol. In the early days, I was too quick to give shoulder pats, even hugs; I wanted to "make it all better" with pep talks and extensions on assignments. The result was a destabilized teacher-student relationship. By now, I'm slightly wiser: I remind myself that I'm a mentor, not a mother; an authority figure, but not authoritarian; someone supportive who maintains a usefully sympathetic distance. I must be interested enough to find out what's wrong, but not so personally involved that I will jeopardize my future effectiveness when stern commentary is warranted.

By now, I know better than to confess my own secret: that I've struggled with depression since 1982, learning (and relearning) to manage what Kurt Vonnegut called "bad chemistry," what Winston Churchill called "The Black Dogs." By now, I've come to regard my own particular dark mongrel almost fondly: as an unsolicited mutt whose erratic behaviour I'll just have to tolerate. And I'm clear that the vagaries of my own mental health fall into the TMI category—too much information—for a student-teacher interaction.

"Kate, can you tell me what's wrong?"

She looks up, gulps, shakes her head. The rim of her brown acrylic turtleneck sweater has been soaking up her tears, and she reaches for a handful of tissue. Her words tumble out in a quavering voice: "I can't do my work . . . I don't care about stuff anymore . . . I don't want to go to class . . . I don't see any point to aaaaanything." More sobs, punctuated by honks into the wad of tissue.

I put my elbows on my knees, lean in closer. "Do you think you might be depressed?"

She shakes her head again, delicate silver-chain earrings trembling in her lobes.

"And maybe that's why you feel so discouraged?"

More sobs, and, finally, a shuddering nod.

Hers seems to be the mood-plunge story all right, the standard version for someone waylaid by depression. But, as always, a few individual facts emerge: she's often felt a bit "down," but never this bad; she thought she could juggle full-time classes with working three nights a week at a café downtown. She started out "pumped" about her studies, but now she can't drag herself out of bed in the morning, much less out of the house, for a 9:30 AM political science class. And her boyfriend is "sick of her moods."

As she talks, she shoots me furtive glances, her voice flat, her eyes bloodshot from tears. She's mortified: crying in front of a professor is *so not cool*.

"Believe me, Kate, this happens to lots of people. Maybe we should call over to Student Health and get you an appointment?"

She blinks, resistant, but willing to be convinced.

"I'll walk over with you, if you want."

■ ■ ■

"Come on, time to get up. You have to get dressed for Group."

I raise my eyelids stealthily, akin to a grave robber prying open a crypt. Fluorescent lights assault me from the ceiling, as if the early-April light bouncing off the remnants of snow is not glaring enough. Wool stuffing muzzles my brain, which nevertheless wants to bust out of my skull. From somewhere at the pit of the fleece, I dredge up the same thought as yesterday and the day before and the day before that: "Shit. I'm awake."

From the hospital corridor, I hear the rattle of the breakfast food wagons, the muted *skreek* of nurses' rubber-soled shoes on marmoleum, the ring-ring of the phone at the nursing station. Worst of all, I smell the fuggy odour of breakfast cooked in advance and kept warm too long on steam trays.

This one is not at all the Big Nurse type. She's a mite of a thing with ropey arms, freckled skin, and curly reddish hair tied at the nape of her neck with a black scarf. She draws back the bedside curtains with a sharp flick of her wrist. As my cotton walls rattle toward the head of my bed, she grabs my right foot through the covers and gives it a hard wobble, like it's a dusty rag she's compelled to shake.

I struggle to sit up, to get a glimpse of her as she swoops toward the door. Here at the University of Alberta Hospital psychiatric ward, no one on staff wears a uniform, as if street clothing will jolly patients along to an early recovery, or at least to a less supine position in bed. Today, Little Nurse pairs khaki pants with an aqua shirt printed with pink hibiscus-like flowers; maybe we'll all be flying to Hawaii later for a midnight luau? Her shoes, though, are sensible beige lace-ups, all the better to creep up on us slothful wretches.

Not only does UAH command its on-duty staff to wear street clothes, it also inflicts the same rules on all its psych patients. I have to get out of bed every morning. And I have to get showered and dressed. No schlumping around in my sleep shirt and flip-flops: I must be up and decent in time for the group (I think of it as the gripe) counselling session—even though I always try to sneak back to bed before lunch.

My back aches and my neck is sore, maybe because I sleep in a tight fetal ball these days, with my chin tucked down to my neck, my knees pulled up to nudge my breasts. I always face the wall to my left, with my back to the patient on my right. She's a teeny, high-strung bulimic who thinks I envy her site beside the window. She's so wrong: lumpen, sunk in my private misery, I'm relieved the empty beige wall reflects nothing back to me, gives me no glimpse of outside life.

■ ■ ■

I don't see Kate for two weeks, so I can only hope for the best. A week after our stroll to Student Health Services, I send her a neutral e-mail that says, "Thinking about you, hope you are doing better." I don't expect a reply. None comes.

■ ■ ■

Memory—or lack thereof—becomes my biggest impediment when I try to look back on that preposterous, horrifying time of my "nervous breakdown." If they are honest, people who suffer from chronic depression will confess to chunks of missing memory in addition to blurred or skewed perceptions about many crucial events. This is especially true if they have ever sought relief by swallowing antidepressants. So, when We the Depressed talk about our illnesses, we seldom deliver a linear chronology. Instead, we stumble on the details, we offer stories with gaps, we have trouble dredging up our doctors' names. Entire key scenarios from our past have gone missing, and we cobble together facts from others' stories. Many of us have shadow memories of free-floating anguish, an actual pain in the head we are only too happy to have dulled by the "meds," of which there is an endless stream for us to test.

"Everybody reacts differently," the doctors say when we ask about the side effects of the latest selective serotonin reuptake inhibitors, known in the trade as SSRIS. "We'll just have to wait and see how you do."

I used to be able to recite reams of poetry from memory; now I can retrieve only snatches. Ironically, I'm chronically unable to remember the names of the antidepressants I have taken over the years, most especially *while I am taking them*. Now, for instance, I'm ingesting something my GP calls . . . pause for memory prod here . . . Pristiq, which sounds to me like either a luxury car or a cut-rate condom. Drugs in the SSRI class include chemical creations such as citalopram, fluoxetine, fluvoxamine, paroxetine, desvenlafaxine, and sertraline. You civilians might be more familiar with their respective trade names: Celexa, Prozac, Luvox, Paxil, Pristiq, and Zoloft. "Flying with Captain Zoloft," a friend of mine joked a while ago, and I knew he wasn't talking about a new airline.

Lacuna: Hiatus, blank, missing portion (especially in ancient manuscript, book, etc.), empty part, cavity in bone, tissue, etc. [Latin = pool, from *lacus* 'lake']
—*The Concise Oxford Dictionary*

So, *lacunae*, plural, *blanks*. I envision my own memory gaps as jagged Swiss-cheese holes poked in the pinky-grey folds of my brain; facts have dropped away into some unfathomable cavern, perhaps never again to be retrieved, no matter how many buckets I hopefully lower on tentative ropes. And yet I draw comfort from the Latin roots of the word; they impart an antiquarian gravitas to that jumbled time in my mid-thirties when I spent six weeks (Or was it eight? No, I checked: one month and two weeks) cocooned in the hospital, lulled by pills and stultifying routines. Midway through my stay, I surfaced enough to realize how truly *grateful* I was to have been advised to commit myself to the psych ward. Being hospitalized gave me permission to stop trying to cope; it forced me to accept help; it gave me a safe place to psychologically "deconstruct."

And, even though, as I started to get better, I chafed against the hospital's rules, resented the group therapy, and had a yelling match with one of the aggressive male nurses who took exception to my insomniac midnight rambles, those institutional routines worked. Gradually, my mood stabilized. Slowly, I began to understand how prolonged, unmediated stress had affected the workings of my brain.

■　■　■

On the third Monday following Kate's tearful session in my office, an envelope arrives through campus mail. A form letter from Kate's counsellor confirms she's suffering from stress-induced depression and is also seeing her MD for "related health issues." She'll need an academic concession to free her from class deadlines until she is better, which might be one month or six months from now. I sign the form with a sense of relief, hoping she'll get the help she needs.

■　■　■

Hunkered down inside the curtains encircling my bed, I skulk behind a towering wall of books. The hard-back edifice stretches across the roll-up bed table where I'm supposed to eat my meals.

When I lie flat on my back, visitors cannot see me from the doorway that opens on to the hospital corridor. My protectors John Peter (*Vladimir's Carrot*), Michel Foucault (*Madness and Civilization*), Hannah Arendt (*The Life of the Mind*), John Berger (*Ways of Seeing*), Laurence Sterne (*The Life and Opinions of Tristram Shandy, Gentleman*) hide me. They are buttressed on either edge of the table by two thick black texts on depression that I checked out of the psychology section of the campus library one day when I was out of the ward on a three-hour pass.

When I tell my psychiatrist I'm a manic-depressive, he bridles. "Who told you *that*?"

Truth is, nobody has. But I've read snatches here and there in those psych texts: "exhausting cycles of energetic flurry followed by abject collapse" exactly describes my life over the past several years. When I am not feeling ashamed that I've fallen apart, I feel relieved to have self-diagnosed my condition. Even if I'm wrong, I need to name my crazy behaviour. Sometimes, late at night, I turn on my bedside lamp and scan the psych texts where I have discovered two memorable new phrases: *exogenous depression, endogenous depression*. The former arises from an external stress or trauma such as a job loss or the death of a loved one. The latter arises without an external identifiable cause and is attributed to chemical imbalance. The former is short term; the latter is chronic or lifelong. (Since then, of course I have looked these phrases up on the Internet again.)

Exogenous/endogenous: the terms comfort me. But I'm also obsessed about the cause of my state: am I suffering from an internal imbalance (was that irascible moodiness of my ancestors actually repressed depression?) or an external precipitating factor (my marriage crashed to bits, and I've survived an unwise love affair)? Have immutable internal factors (inherited murky-brain chemistry) or external events (a thesis focused on post-modern instability) caused me to crack up? In short, *is my depression an innie or an outie*? I have not yet read enough to know how sly the brain can be, how treacherous the pas de deux between stress and brain chemistry. And I'm appalled to learn that even the doctors don't seem to know how to differentiate causal factors—or how to tell the endogenous and exogenous depressions apart. *Oh, that's just great: so I can be depressed from two separate causes simultaneously and can't tell which one has me in its clutches?*

The truth is, my book fortress provides dubious comfort: I struggle daily to read at least part of a chapter but feel increasingly frantic when I cannot remember anything—not even if I reread the same page five times in a row. Nevertheless, I keep my BookWall intact: I want to believe it tells everyone I am more than just the dead-eyed zombie they see in this bed, more than just another crazy in a four-bed room. My BookWall fibs to everyone for me, but in my occasional lucid moments, I realize how preposterous it looks to visitors, how annoying it is to the nurses trying to care for me, how pathetic the psychiatrists must find it.

Later, much later, I will understand that some ragtag remnant of my previous personality insisted on my childish book barricade because I thought it announced that, in my "real life" outside the psych ward, I was something other than a condition: I was a struggling thinker, a muddled student of literature, a good cook and gregarious friend, an *actual person*.

For the first two or three weeks on the ward, I carom between waterworks and oblivion. I wake up and sob. The nurses give me two blue (or were they yellow?) pills. I swallow. I'm slugged back into sleep. In five or six hours I awaken and cry again. The nurses dole out more pills. Blessed obliteration resumes.

■　■　■

I have to confess that I don't remember much about my initial "breakdown." It seems ludicrous to admit that my collapse started just after my 10:00 AM coffee break when Sally/Sarah pranced past my office. When we all began the doctoral program in English, she'd been Sally, but apparently a numerologist had said her name projected bad vibes. So she became Sarah. We thought this was ridiculous, so we called her *Sally/Sarah* behind her back.

"So, how's your thesis going?" S/S had asked that morning, stopping a couple feet past my doorway. I harbour a hazy picture of her tucking a few stray strands of blond hair behind her ears as she stood there.

I must have gawped at her as if she were speaking in tongues. "Ah, ahh, aaaaah," I answered. Or something like that. Then I slammed the door and dissolved on the floor. My thesis? Of course, my thesis was not "going." Or coming. Not at all. Naught. I was stuck, marooned, stranded, unable to think or write, and the stasis was driving me crazy.

Apparently, I was still there on the floor much later, snivelling and hiccoughing. Not acceptable academic behaviour. Then my friend Candace arrived to walk me across campus to the hospital's Emergency Room. Years later, she told me that I kept yammering that jumping off the High Level Bridge was a viable solution to my misery. People still entertain that idea—and a few of them are fatally successful each year.

"I kept thinking I could tackle you, if you tried to make a run for it," she recalled.

■ ■ ■

When I grope backwards over several decades, I realize that I have packed away several memories of student suicides. The worst occurred in the mid-1970s at the University of Lethbridge during a Christmas break when a student hanged herself under the student residence that overlooked the Oldman River. Rumour was, she was not found for several days. It took everyone a long time to shake off that guilt. I can only hope that Kate has not been driven to such extremes, but I have no access to any reassuring information.

■ ■ ■

After I checked out of the university hospital and went back to my cramped apartment, I had to consign myself to mandatory psychotherapy four mornings a week. For a while, I personified the term *lachrymally labile*. I continued to weep in Dr. L's office, but only for fifty minutes at a time. Gradually, I came to see that I had been teetering on a steep bank for a long time before Sally/Sarah's question pushed me into the torrent that swirled me beyond any coherent shore. Finally, I understood how dangerous my own little self-created Petri dish had become: not sleeping for weeks was abnormal; racketing through my low-rent apartment, rigid with anxiety, was a sure guarantee that I'd never complete any academic work; full-blown task avoidance was patently unhealthy—though common—graduate student behaviour. In time, I could actually laugh at myself as I told Dr. L how I drank a bottle of cooking sherry one dark desperate night; how, to occupy my twitchy hands, I chomped through several five-pound sacks of Macintosh apples a week. "I have heard of worse addictions," he said, making only the briefest note on my little manias.

■　■　■

It's September again. Wraiths of early-morning fog waft through Mount Douglas Park as I drive to work. For the past few weeks, activity on campus has quickened: the library is busy again, more bodies stroll the paths, guitar-strumming students gather by the Petch Fountain. For me, the calendar year always begins in September, never in January. September means a new term, a new set of classes, a whole new series of beginnings. Today is the first day of my second-year writing workshop, and I scan the course list as I begin roll call, noting new people, recognizing others from last semester.

My eyes skid to a halt. I look up: there she is, whispering something to the student next to her, then laughing. She's cut her hair short and spiky, and her skin is tanned golden brown.

"Kate," I say. "Nice to see you again."

The Biology of
Human Starvation

LAURA INGRAM

This disease, it sounds like teeth, chattering inside my chapped skull. While I shiver on my friend's bedroom floor, she brings me a Dixie cup full of lukewarm water, brushes some brittle baby hairs off my forehead.

"You are the skinniest girl in the world!" She cries over my moth-eaten bones for four hours. Her words can't quite reach me. It's as if I've already died.

Nervosa started like a false alarm, something set for another dawn, something I should have ignored. I was sixteen and in my sophomore year. My hipbones felt sharper than before and when I looked in the mirror, my light-bulb ilium flickered behind my lantern-paper skin. Starving was like getting my prescription for my glasses tweaked — I walked with more purpose, sure I could see the fashioning of an unclaimed future further ahead without bothering to look both ways. I had no need to be a role model anymore.

"Laura, please. Get up."

When my best friend and I babysit her little brother, he always offers me the half of the Oreo with icing, never asks if he can sit in my lap. While I slip my shoes back on at the end of the day, he tugs on her sleeve, asks if I weigh half of what he does.

He is seven years old.

Whenever I get home from a friend's house or school or a walk my parents want to know what I ate, but even a carton of juice to stop the shakes makes my amygdala itch. I swallow hard, ashamed.

My skin has been replaced with freezer burn, my insides with dry rot. My teeth are the cold snap that stunts the Baby's Breath in the flowerbed out back. I am in the throes of a chill, arthritic as autumn, a pavement of primary colour. People who don't understand the science of decay think it's a beautiful thing; that as the archeologist of my own skeleton, plucking my sternum out of the ash, I have given them a primary source for the analysis of eternity.

But where is this beauty? There is a boy who rubs my knuckles where they rust for luck. My hair still falls out and my skirt swings more than it should. I pin it to my pelvic bone, step out of it without unzipping it to stand on the scale. The scale counts backwards like an anaesthesiologist, the numbers getting lower until I sleep without feeling the shiver of the antiseptic, without knowing where the surgeon will slice.

■   ■   ■

Sometimes when I come home from school, my legs bow out beneath me. The contraction is out of my control; this is more a matter of efficacy than anything else. Origami, after all, is an art form.

I don't consider it contortion.

The trouble is I can never quite remember how to unfold.

My mother says clean your plate. My father says just a little more. My sister doesn't say anything.

I don't remember the first time I slipped on the slick bottom of my shower, holding onto my hipbones, convinced that all the dirt in these coordinates on the prime meridian had been crushed beneath my eyelids. Full of groundwater and a heart like a mosquito, buzzing and bumping dumbly.

No matter how much I scrubbed my skin, scoured my teeth, straightened up the crawlspaces between my bones, I felt like my body was a haunted house, not the right place for me to grow up, full of other people's dust.

It really started at age nine and a half. I had squeaky shoes and a squeaky voice. I read three chapter books a week and I threw my peanut butter sandwiches in the garbage every day, untouched, on the way to recess.

My two best friends teased me, skinny minnie, mosquito legs. But I'd always been skinny; five pounds at birth, fifty on my tenth birthday.

Nobody noticed me crumbling my cake into the lace-edged napkin on my lap before I tried to blow the trick candles out.

■ ■ ■

I was a long-boned eleven, listless and lithe. Rigor mortis starts at the shins: the other kids stared, and I stopped, knowing God was not as near as I'd always thought. The sixth-grade locker room smelled like peanut butter and Powder Fresh. We turned our attention away from each other and towards the hooks and straps of our new training bras.

"Oh my god, look how skinny she is." They nudged each other with scabby elbows, and I wrapped my arms around my ribcage.

"Do you like, eat? Ever?" I stared at the scuffmarks on my sequined sneakers, jerked my shirt over my head. Glitter eye shadow smeared my glasses.

"Of course I do. All the time."

It wasn't a lie. I had breakfast every morning before the bus came, because I'd read in some magazine my mother kept on the coffee table that kids who don't eat breakfast are more likely to become overweight. There were just lots of foods that skimmed my stomach like dull scissors. I didn't like to eat as much as they did, didn't need to.

I stomped up the stoop stairs after school, cried with my fists closed and my bedroom door open. My mother's palm startled me from half-sleep hours later.

"Dinner's ready," she said. I bit my bottom lip.

"I'm not hungry yet."

■ ■ ■

Sixty-nine pounds of glitter and mace, grade eight came like a single session of electroshock therapy, short-circuited my eye sockets.

The other kids called me Little Auschwitz, made gagging sounds whenever I asked a teacher for the bathroom pass. In gym class, even the smaller boys picked me up and moved me if they felt I was in their way.

My phone was always seizing in ringtone with acrid messages from people whose floors I'd built blanket forts on, whose bowling birthday parties I'd been invited to back in the sixth and seventh grades:

"You look like you're dying, you're either seven or seventy."

"If I have a baby and it weighs less than three pounds I'll be sure to name it after you."

"You must shop in the toddler's section, they don't make skinny jeans skinny enough for you, go buy a goddamn glitter belt at the kid's clothing store."

"How many times a day do you puke, what the hell is wrong with you anyway—?"

I slipped my training bra off in front of the bathroom mirror, let my denim skirt pool around my ankles, traced my twitching fingers over my bones as they bent their softened heads in defeat. Infrastructure almost always crumbles during overexposure.

I wished I could slip back inside the red clay that preceded original sin, thin as a rib, safe under the arm of another.

Or maybe I was inherently flawed before the bite.

Either way, nothing was enough.

■ ■ ■

I'm still on my friend's bedroom floor. Tucking my hair behind my ears, I try to stand. My limbs feel like they have been borrowed from another body. I go to the Governor's School now, for fine arts and fine lines, and no one makes fun of me. Instead they cup their hands over their clicking teeth as if they are trying to cover something contagious. Even now, some are still superstitious enough to keep away from my corpse.

My parents have started making me sit at the table. I stir some tomatoes and vinegar with my fork, pray for the apocalypse of my carotid artery as I stare at the Tiffany lamp swaying on the swirl ceiling.

"You can't stay alive long at this weight. It's either eat or go to the hospital."

My esophagus shivers, and I swallow some of the auburn slime off my fork, choke on a seed.

"It's my body." My hands shake, but my voice steadies. "I destroy it."

My parents slump forward in their chairs, elbows on the table. I'm not the only one who has lost interest in what is right.

■　■　■

Frail as last Friday's cigarette papers, I am crumpled into the back seat of my mother's car. The hospital encroaches in a city the colour of a heart-attack victim's face, kept alive by the constant click and murmur of machines. We measure its pulse in miles per hour, starting and stopping like an arrhythmia.

A young nurse who pops her gum and snaps her fingers comes in to give me an EKG. I shimmy out of my tank top.

"Oh, you are so lucky to be sooo skinny! I bet you can wear anything you want!"

The only things that fit me at this point are skirts made for seven-year-olds. I cringe. By now I know that EKGs don't hurt, but the table is cold and my vertebrae roll around on it like marbles.

My parents take me to my favourite restaurant when the tests are done. I stare at the California rolls, bite my lip until blood comes, fish a gel pen out of my purse. My friend had turned away from me in tears the week before, and she's stopped picking up the phone when I call, so I write her a note on a napkin.

Please remember me as stronger than I seem and just as graceful as you think.

The ink smudges where the punctuation is supposed to be.

Tomorrow, I am going to another hospital. One for people like me who search their throats with two fingers for the hollow that gets sore just before the cigarette, who hunger and are left dissipating and disappointed.

When we get up to take the check to the front, I grab a couple of pieces of candy from the basket by the till.

My parents cradle me by my scapula, catching scraps of shoulder blade between their swerving fingers.

This is how we say goodbye, again and again, pretending not to know.

Rainy Day

CLARISSA HART

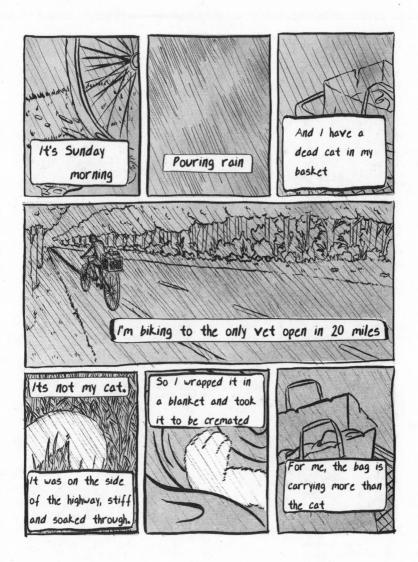

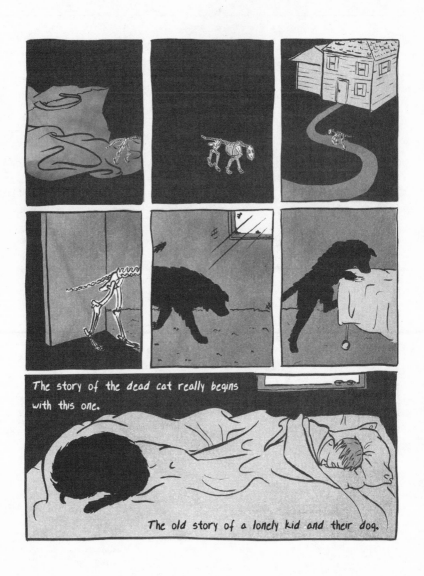

The story of the dead cat really begins with this one.

The old story of a lonely kid and their dog.

As a kid, a vindictive world is better than indifference. Even if the world was cruel, at least it was paying attention.

And I could try to figure out the rules and avoid the world's punishment. Two I figured out early: be quiet, and stay alone.

I was afraid, not of being hurt, but of hurting other people. I thought something in me was rotten or poisonous, or I was just too clumsy and strange to ever belong.

But I thought a dog would be safe

I knew getting attached to something was a transgression, but he was alone like I was, only he didn't mind. I had a friend, so I minded less, too.

When he starved to death. I took it hard, because it was my fault.

I'd broken the rules.

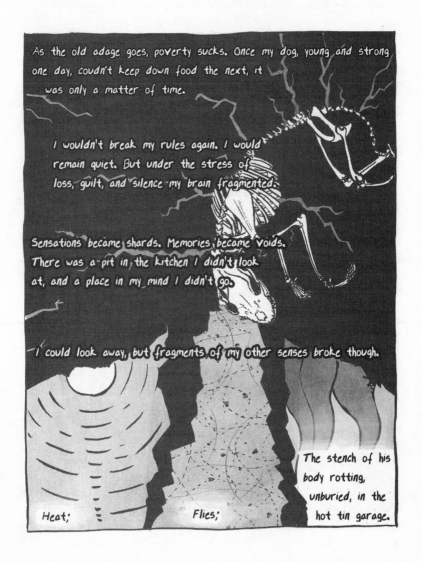

As the old adage goes, poverty sucks. Once my dog, young and strong one day, couldn't keep down food the next, it was only a matter of time.

I wouldn't break my rules again. I would remain quiet. But under the stress of loss, guilt, and silence my brain fragmented.

Sensations became shards. Memories became voids. There was a pit in the kitchen I didn't look at, and a place in my mind I didn't go.

I could look away, but fragments of my other senses broke though.

Heat;

Flies;

The stench of his body rotting, unburied, in the hot tin garage.

That's how my thoughts for years, pieces rather than a narrative. There were things I skipped over like jumping over cracks in ice. But some things pulled me in.

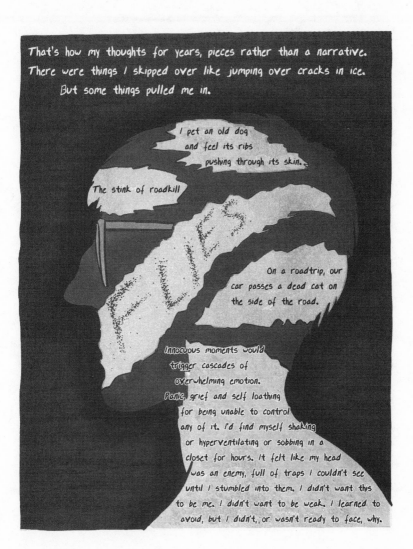

I pet an old dog and feel its ribs pushing through its skin.

The stink of roadkill

On a roadtrip, our car passes a dead cat on the side of the road.

Innocuous moments would trigger cascades of overwhelming emotion. Panic, grief and self loathing for being unable to control any of it. I'd find myself shaking or hyperventilating or sobbing in a closet for hours. It felt like my head was an enemy, full of traps I couldn't see until I stumbled into them. I didn't want this to be me. I didn't want to be weak. I learned to avoid, but I didn't, or wasn't ready to face, why.

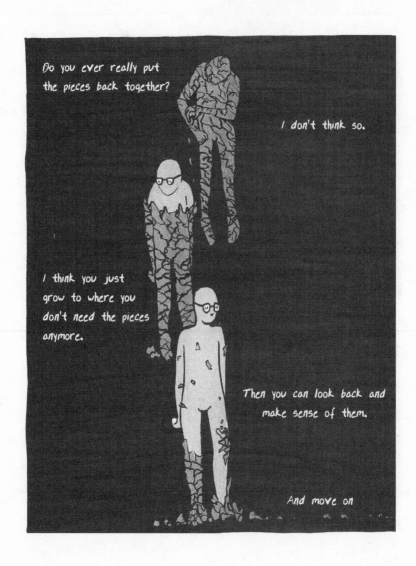

You live life in instances. Not the long succession of years and therapy, but the moments when you show yourself you've changed.

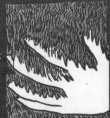

Years later, as a volunteer at a pet clinic, I'd hold animals left by their owners to be euthanized. Because I didn't want to be the coward who let them die alone.

And in this moment, inches away from a dead cat in a bag, who's it for. The cat, past caring, to prove the world isn't as negligent as it seems.

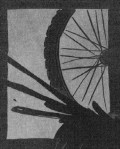

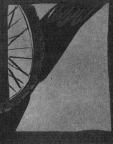

For my dog, in hopes of an atonement I don't deserve.

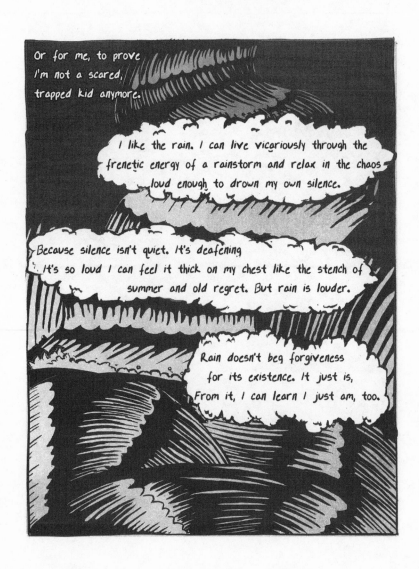

My Brother, My Sister

In a Quiet Room

ANDREW BODEN

In April 1997, when my brother's life fell apart for the third time, visitors entered Royal Columbian's Psychiatric Emergency Department through a thick teal door to the left of the main entrance. There was a makeshift waiting room before the teal door, which had four black vinyl chairs and a pine coffee table on which lay a stack of three-year-old *Maclean's* and *Sports Illustrated* magazines. A stencilled sign above the door, which was always closed, read, *Psychiatric Emergency* in black letters and there were no instructions what to do—wait or knock or phone—no one to receive you as there was for physical injuries at the Emergency Department twenty feet across the hall. Noise poured from Emergency: the chatter of nurses and doctors, the thump and squeak of shoes, the low hum of gurney wheels on the floor; there were cries and groans and, from the reception desk, how-may-I-help-you's. Not a sound came from behind the thick teal door of the Psychiatric Emergency Department.

This was my first of too many visits here and I didn't know the door was locked. I tugged on the door handle, and when it didn't give I threw a bewildered look at the Emergency Department, where patients and nurses went in and out without care. The receptionist in Emergency told me that I had to knock—"Knock loud or they won't hear ya!" I rapped on the heavy door. I waited for a count of twenty and then rapped again.

The door opened four or five inches on a thick-chested man in a short-sleeved white shirt and a black tie, a weary-looking security guard from the Paladin Security Company.

"I'm here to see my brother," I said.

He closed the door to confirm my story with a nurse. Two minutes passed, then three, then ten. I began to wonder if I should sit down again or knock a third time or just go the hell home. Finally, he let me in. The door swung shut behind me. The latch clicked as it locked. I might have called the silence in that room calm or meditative, if I didn't know that it had been achieved with powerful drugs, the heavy tranquilizers the pharmaceutical industry rebranded as antipsychotics. There was a high, teal-veneer desk where a nurse wrote on a clipboard and, to the right, a row of three closed doors at intervals of fifteen feet. Each door was baby-pink and as thick as the one I had come through and each one had a small central window, about the size of a hardcover novel, which was hinged so that it could be opened from the outside.

I gave the RN my name and told him that I was here to see my brother who had been sent here by Dr. M, his psychiatrist at Tri-Cities Mental Health.

"You don't want to see your brother right now," the nurse said. "Come back tomorrow."

"My brother should see someone he knows," I insisted. Or used to know or pretended to know because by then the lives of J and I had irrevocably divided. I went to university and graduated and he went to university but didn't graduate because his panic attacks grew too severe and so began his slow spiral into places I didn't want to go.

I wanted, however, to comfort him. He had a live-in girlfriend, at least for a few months longer, but few friends and even fewer old friends once they met his schizophrenia in person. And he'd arrived at Royal Columbian earlier in the afternoon not in the back of an ambulance, as he thought Dr. M meant when she said he could be escorted to the hospital for a second opinion, but in the back of a police car with three RCMP officers. When he arrived, six security guards made him surrender his clothes and possessions and escorted him into one of the three "seclusion rooms," as the hospital staff called these cells.

J must have seen or heard me because he edged toward the little window in the door. The security guard gave me a weary look, as if he knew how this was going to end, and loomed just out of J's sight.

"Five minutes," the RN said to me. He didn't open the door to my brother's cell. J and I had to talk through the Plexiglas window set in the door.

My brother's beautiful face, the same beautiful face for which girls once followed him home from his lifeguard job at the swimming pool, was pale and gaunt, a flimsy thing discarded and picked up again and again no matter how ill it began to fit. His eyes blazed like little searchlights I wanted to turn away from.

"I don't know why I'm here," J said.

"I don't know either," I replied. I forced myself not to cry. "I'll talk to Dr. M first thing tomorrow."

My brother nodded and shuffled away from the window. He wore only a loose-fitting light blue hospital gown that was open at the back and would've better fit a man two sizes smaller. I could see the shallow furrow of his spine down to his buttocks. He shrank into the far corner, my six-foot-four brother, shrank to his haunches and wrapped a second gown around his eyes and wept.

■ ■ ■

The next morning at the Tri-Cities Mental Health Centre, I couldn't see Dr. M or J's regular psychiatric nurse. I spoke to a second nurse, Jack, who told me that Dr. M certified J as delusional with no insight into his condition and a danger to himself and society. I said that I didn't understand why J, who had never been violent despite his outbursts, had to be locked in a cell.

"There is no other procedure," Jack said, "to treat cases like your brother. Everyone in his condition goes to the seclusion room. It's pathetic and inhumane and you should write the Hospital Board about it."

J's "seclusion room" at Royal Columbian was twelve feet by twelve feet between four baby pink walls and the only furnishings were a single mattress on the floor, an "anti-suicide" toilet bolted to the opposite wall, and a red panic button near the door. My brother told me later that he thought of the room as a puzzle he had to solve to escape. If he could line up the bank of fluorescent lights, the red button, and the toilet, and when all the pieces fit just right, the door would pop open and he could escape. But the nurses and the doctors always interrupted his attempts to solve the room, he said, with pills or food or "stupid ass" questions. The shrinks, he said, came around at 6:00 AM before they drove their Mercedes to their suburban practices.

When I returned to the Psychiatric Emergency that afternoon, the nurses had left my brother's cell door open—an order from his psychiatrist, who came and went like a phantom. J lay cocooned in two layers of hospital sheets. The fluorescent lights hummed. The room smelled of a powerful, sweet disinfectant. I edged over the threshold and waited for the cell door to slam shut behind me as if I'd walked into a giant Venus flytrap.

I knelt beside J's immobile form and struggled against my reserved nature to reach out for his hand. He looked placid, better than the previous day, a man saved from a hurricane, battered but not drowned. The drugs had worked; I thought they had worked. I believed in the system, I believed in a straight, unswerving path to mental health.

■　■　■

Three days after my brother's admission, I stood with him and his girlfriend, Angela, in the hazy sunshine as he smoked outside the main entrance. The psychiatrists had prescribed him loxapine, an antipsychotic to treat his delusions, sleeplessness, incoherent speech, and excessive aggression. The staff moved him out of his seclusion room and gave him a bed in the Emergency Department. More privileges followed, such as smoking outside and wearing street clothes, as patients, theoretically, grew well.

My brother told me that one of the volunteers, a man who showed him how to play Chinese Poker, worked for a firm that researched methane fuel cells. J said as far as technology was concerned humanity should slow down. I asked what he meant. He said that we shouldn't regard this as psychotic, but if aliens were watching the Earth they might be getting upset.

"I'm not saying that there are aliens," he added, "but if you saw a country progressing faster than you, wouldn't you get pissed off?"

He grew frustrated with my questions and said it was just an analogy and wanted to go back inside. He lay back down on his narrow bed and swore at us and mocked Angela. I confided to a nurse that J was still saying bizarre things and acting aggressively toward his girlfriend. She said that the doctor had noted this and would be seeing him at 2:00 PM. I told Angela what I'd said and she agreed with me. I left for home thinking my brother was in good hands.

I phoned Psychiatric Emergency several times and several times I waited on hold for what seemed like hours and, finally, at 6:00 PM, I learned that J had been discharged by a different psychiatrist, Dr. O, a man I'd never met and who had never tried to contact me about J's state of mind. He had diagnosed J with "marijuana psychosis," which was a new addition to the growing laundry list of disorders my brother had been labelled with: bipolar, schizophrenia, schizoaffective, still more I couldn't recall.

I phoned J at his home. I said I was worried for him. He said that he could prove everyone was crazy anyway, so what did his mind matter to me? I said that he was still having bizarre thoughts and wasn't well.

"Like how?" he snapped.

I mentioned his concern that some unknown "they" could clone our dead father from his teeth. I mentioned the scene on Sunday, when he squatted on the ground outside the hospital and picked through bits of debris and put a bit of foil and a tiny chunk of glass in his pocket.

"I was looking for a weapon," J said.

"You told me to worship pagan gods," I replied.

"They're better than the Christian one. Besides, who's crazy? Me or the brother who brought me a Fred Saberhagen novel to read in the mental ward?"

I called Dr. O's office repeatedly. I left dozens of messages. He never phoned me back. I gave up too easily. I prayed my brother was taking his medication. He wasn't. He came by my apartment two days later to return one of my books. He didn't trust the psychiatrists, he said, and blew off the three medications they had prescribed him. He said I should be wary of leaving genetic traces lying around, because "they" could get them. I didn't know what to do. Everyone in this crazy cycle thought they knew what to do: my brother, the psychiatrists, the pharmaceutical companies, me in my moments of certainty after I read this or that book on the brain or schizophrenia or psychotherapy. Our vanities, our seductive vanities, went undiagnosed and untreated as the circus wheel went around and around.

■ ■ ■

Three days later at ten in the morning, I knocked on the door of my brother's basement suite to help he and Angela move. J, Angela said, had stormed off to the gas station in his bathrobe to fill a jerry can for his Toyota MR2, and when he returned, he roared off without out telling her where he was going. He'd raged and stormed before I'd arrived and upturned their bedroom and the packing boxes full of the things we were supposed to move to their new place in Port

Coquitlam. We talked about what to do: wait for him to come back or phone the police or . . . ? I didn't want to phone the police again, I didn't want my brother dragged back into a cell. Angela went to pick up my youngest brother, S, because we didn't have enough help now that J had left. My wife told me on the phone to call the police. I wandered around their apartment struggling to find a phone book in the carnage, so I could call the RCMP's non-emergency number, take a half-measure I wouldn't feel as terrible about. I phoned my wife for the non-emergency number. She told me to call 911.

I explained J's condition to the 911 operator, my worries for him, my worries about the system, the cells in the Psychiatric Emergency, the debilitating antipsychotics, the hospital psychiatrist who had swooped in like a bungling, absentee father to fix everything. "Everything is going to work out," the operator reassured me. "Try not to overthink it."

I wandered around J and Angela's apartment again. I didn't know what to do, so I began to load their things into the truck. An RCMP patrol car roared up minutes later, and right in front of my brother's landlord, I had to explain what happened, my brother's psychological state, his recent time in Royal Columbian. The constable issued an APB on the spot through his radio and gave me a case file number on his card. The landlord began to tell the constable every miserable thing he could think of about J and Angela. I couldn't listen. I went back to putting their things into the truck and worried that my brother would race up in his car in god knows what deranged state.

The police phoned me at 2:00 PM. They'd found my brother wandering around at Barnet and Lougheed, searching for a nonexistent missing girl. He was showing everyone he met one of Angela's baby pictures—the missing girl.

■ ■ ■

I sat on the floor beside my brother in a second Seclusion Room at Royal Columbian. He sobbed. He said something happened to his car. It wouldn't start, so he abandoned it. I found his MR2 an hour later where he left it under the overpass on Front Street in New Westminster. The driver's side door was wide open and the interior light glowed dimly. There were two cans of Friskies cat food in a white plastic bag on top of the roof. The interior was a mess of cigarette ash and garbage, but it still smelled like my father: sweet sweat, cedar, and lanolin. The car had been our father's divorce gift to himself before he died nine months earlier. It was my father who looked after my brother the first time he fell apart, who held his hand when J's muscles went taunt and rigid from the first anti-psychotics, who never forgave himself for the emotional damage he felt he inflicted on his second son. I shifted the car into park from reverse and it started immediately.

J was moved into SC2 in the Sherbrooke Psychiatric Facility a few days later. SC2 remained as eerily quiet as the Psychological Emergency was when I first arrived. Patients shuffled around the floor in blue gowns or street clothes when they had re-earned the right to wear them. The nurses sat behind their station in a cloud of boredom and spoke in low voices or flipped through magazines until the next dispensation of medication. Here any emotion outside the reserved Canadian norm was considered abnormal. Garden-variety anger attracted RNs with a lecture or Ativan or the threat of a visit to the Quiet Room, Sherbrooke's version of the seclusion room.

My daily visits to see J blurred together. One day his medication made him anxious and we marched up and down the hallway, which had a sign at either end that read, *80 laps makes one kilometre. Go for it!* Every few minutes J dropped to the floor and pumped out push-ups because the anxiety from his meds, he said, "drives me fucking crazy." He complained to the nurses, but they insisted that this side effect was much better than psychosis, but didn't explain for whom. Another day, my brother wore a plastic, fluorescent cross and called himself by his middle name, Michael, because he believed he was the Archangel Michael. Our father, he confided in me, was in Hell. Every lap, up or down the floor, we walked past a large, sky blue construction paper collage of the fun activities patients could amuse themselves with on the ward. The collage didn't say that the only game on the common room computer was Doom, which I played when I waited for my brother to come back from group therapy, or *group*, as patients called it. Outside on the front steps my brother chain-smoked, as it seemed every patient at Sherbrooke chain-smoked to cope with madness and its salves.

Eight days after my brother's second admission, his psychiatrist, Dr. O, finally agreed to meet with Angela and me. Dr. O had never answered any of our numerous notes or returned a single one of our phone calls, so the meeting shocked me. We met at 10:00 AM in a conference room with Dr. O, a social worker, and a psychiatric nurse.

Dr. O began the meeting by saying that he hoped we could provide some information that would shed some light on my brother's case.

I said that Angela and I had been struggling to contact him by phone for ten days to tell him just that.

He told us never to phone him at his office.

"How can we contact you?" I asked.

"You may leave a note," he said.

"You never answered any of our notes."

"You may leave a note."

Angela asked numerous questions about my brother's condition and his prognosis, and to each question Dr. O said that my brother had little insight into his condition and likely wouldn't take his medication.

She asked Dr. O about the side effects of loxapine, the antipsychotic he'd prescribed J. He said that drugs like loxapine took two to three weeks to reach useful antipsychotic effect.

"Knowing that," I said at volume, "you discharged my brother into the community with a prescription after only three days in the Emergency Department?"

"What would you have us do?" he asked.

"Admit him and stabilize him on medication."

He dismissed this with a shake of his head.

I grew irate. I said that he'd discharged my brother too early, he'd failed to consult with the family, he failed to return phone calls, he'd strayed from the DSM-IV, the bible of psychiatric diagnosis, by concluding my brother had "marijuana psychosis." I said that I had to phone 911 to get my brother off the street.

Dr. O called this old news and then said to me, "I understand you use marijuana."

"I do not," I said. "And even if I did, what does that have to do with discharging my brother too early?"

He said that according to J and Angela, I shared marijuana with them.

Angela told Dr. O that he had the wrong brother. My youngest brother smoked marijuana with them.

Dr. O muttered, "Oh," but didn't apologize.

By now I was yelling at him, every furious thing I could think to indict the bastard with.

By now the social worker was yelling at me, "We are not mind readers!" and, finally, Dr. O said that if I didn't silence myself he'd have security remove me.

He turned to Angela and said, "Do you have anything reasonable to say?"

■　■　■

My brother later told me that the whole floor on SC2 heard me bawling out Dr. O. "You're lucky," J said, "they didn't lock you in the Quiet Room. Or me, to punish you." I wrote letters to the head of psychiatry, Dr. C. Angela also wrote letters to Dr. C: the psychiatric staff, she wrote, had forced her to take J back to their home; she felt as if she had no choice. Dr. C wrote back. The outcome of the meeting was my own fault: I was angry and belligerent from the start. Dr. O had behaved with patience and professionalism and wasn't, as I described him in my first letter, *dismissive, condescending, supercilious, burdened with excessive professional vanity and completely lacking in professional judgement.* I could have raged about Dr. O to the College of Physicians and Surgeons, but my anger wouldn't have done anything for my brother.

In early September, my brother vanished again for a few days. He lived on Wreck Beach until security guards at the University of British Columbia chased him into the surf. I didn't hesitate to knock on the heavy teal door to the Psychiatric Emergency Department.

This time, I felt like an old veteran.

I spoke in a soft voice.

On the Way to Here

JUDY McFARLANE

The man sits in a dingy white plastic lawn chair facing the high chain-link fence. Ball cap pulled low, he sinks back in the chair, smoking as he stares out across the wide river. On the far side, in the failing light, the smelter glows, plumes of gases, pink, orange, white, venting into the night sky. As I walk toward him, the man half turns, giving me a puzzled look.

"John?"

The man stands up. After a moment, his face splits in a wide grin and he's hugging me, tight and fierce, my face mashed into his smoky shoulder. As he releases me, his grin slides into a sheepish smile. "In the loony bin now," my brother says.

Although he's been here for a month, the doctors can't agree on John's diagnosis. It might be a brain tumour, seizures, a stroke, or syphilis. We sit down beside each other in the faded chairs.

"I've got a few theories," John says. I wait, staring across the river at the brilliant lights of the smelter. His words spit out, as if he's been saving them up for me. "I've got all the numbers on my computer at home, every one she calls, I've figured out the pattern and I can predict which one will be next. It's been going on for a long time, I just didn't see it before, guys I know too." He takes a drag and continues. "I can print it out for you if you want, you want to see it?"

I shake my head. For most of our adult lives, my brother and I have lived four hundred miles apart. Close enough to visit a few times every year but far enough that we don't really know what happens in each other's lives. From a distance, his marriage has seemed stable, as happy as any other long-term marriage.

John doesn't look at me as he talks. I think of him as a young boy, of the excitement that always surrounded him, the sense that anything could happen, that danger swelled just below the surface, ready to crash through into daylight.

■ ■ ■

Shivering, I stand on the veranda with my mother. Behind us hangs the morning's laundry, stiff and heavy. My mother's breath jabs out in sharp, dense clouds as she scans the snowbank beside the road. "John!" she shouts. "Where are you?" All morning, John has been digging new tunnels in the snowbank. Now, the grader is plowing its way up our street. I hold my breath as it passes in front of us, a high arc of snow fanning out from its blade. My mother puts her hand to her mouth and makes a sound, something that's not a word. I squint at the snowbank, trying to control the painful white light it emits. Then, emerging from the light, an arm, a head. My brother, grinning, waving to us.

■ ■ ■

The air is cold and it's quiet now. We can hear the steady rumble of the smelter, a heavy sound punctuated by clanks, thuds, mechanical whooshes.

John lights another cigarette. He doesn't seem to want to go inside, where the door will lock behind him. He turns to me, his cigarette hand tracing a red line. "I've got a plan," he says. "Got a partner too, he's going to bankroll us until the financing comes through. The plan is to subdivide; it's ten acres and we can turn that into one-acre plots and sell them. They'll go like hotcakes!"

I ask John where the property is. He gives me a look that says I've missed the main point. "It's my property, that's the land, I mean." I can't stop myself from staring at him. He lives on a five-acre plot just outside of town. He's worked at a pulp mill all his life. He knows nothing about property development. "You'll see," he says.

■ ■ ■

John races past me, leading a troop of his friends into our second-floor bathroom. I want to ask him what he's doing, but I know when his friends are with him, I'm invisible. I edge forward so I can peek into the bathroom. John is perched on the window ledge. He turns to his friends and says, "If you push hard, like this"—he grips the sides of the narrow window frame—"then you can make it." He pushes off, falling out of sight. His friends squirm forward like puppies and peer down. Silence. I hold my breath. Is John dead in the narrow space between our house and the neighbour's house? Then one friend shouts, and the rest shout too, a happy, raucous sound. The friends swarm past me and down the stairs. I walk into the bathroom and look out the window. Below, on the sloping porch roof of the house next door, John looks up at me, a wide grin on his face.

■ ■ ■

I'm ten years old. I know I should try to stop him. But I want to see what will happen. John has just pulled his best friend's BB gun from under his bed and is pointing it at the house across the street. He leans out his window and squeezes the trigger. A window splits and shatters. John squeezes again and again. The sound of the shattering glass exhilarates me. I feel a heady combination of dread and high excitement. My brother has just blown out all the front windows of the house owned by the school librarian, a stern woman hated by students, a woman my father, also a teacher, calls his colleague.

When my father arrives home that night, I press against the wall as he pushes past me to John's room. I hear his angry voice, followed by a hard smack. Then another and another. When it's silent and my father has gone downstairs, I peer into John's room. He sits cross-legged on his bed, reading a comic. He glances up at me, his cheek bright red. "I don't care," he whispers. "I'm glad I did it."

■　■　■

One morning I drive with John and his wife to see the only neurologist in the area. Her office is an hour's drive away. As my sister-in-law drives, John and I sit in the back seat, John talking as if we're alone. "She won't listen to me, she says I take too long to say anything, I have to be faster. Just get to the end, she says. I can only talk the way I talk. She needs to listen."

John faces the window as he talks, his head turned away from me. I catch my sister-in-law's eye in the rear-view mirror. She gives a slight shrug, as if this is the least of her worries. I suddenly realize that when our mother died a few months ago, John no longer had anyone who would listen. He was on his own.

■　■　■

Sometime past midnight, a small noise wakes me. It's John. I drift back to sleep to the rise and fall of voices, a soft murmur, as John and my mother talk in the kitchen. The next morning, my mother tells me they sat up all night. "What did you talk about?" I ask. "Oh," she says, "everything. He talks and I listen."

As a child, I often resented my mother's attention to John, and what seemed her scattered attention to me. But as a teenager, I began to understand. The high fever of energy I always felt when John was around was now manifesting itself in minor car accidents, failure at school, arriving home so drunk his friends had to carry him. By waiting up for John, by talking him through the night, my mother was doing what she could to ride the turbulence with him, to give him something to hang on to.

■ ■ ■

While the neurologist taps John's knees with her small hammer, I tell her that John looked after our parents in their last years. I mention my mother's cancer, my father's dementia. I don't tell her that John was the person who answered my father's questions over and over, the person who got in his car and went looking when my mother called to say that my father had gone out at three in the morning. I don't mention that John lifted my mother from her wheelchair to the bed when she couldn't walk anymore. But I think about those things and my voice dies. The neurologist looks up at us and says, "I can't find any evidence of damage."

Growing up, I never thought about whether John's ups and downs amounted to an identifiable cluster of characteristics, one that could be labelled and treated. He was my brother, the person who created a space for me, who let me tag along, who never tried to foist blame on me. I realized that he had given me a profound gift: the lucky family position of innocent bystander. While he spun out twin threads of exhilaration and dread, I had a ringside seat, seeing it all, never having to take any responsibility.

The doctors finally decide that my brother has bipolar disorder. Unusual, they tell us, for someone in his late fifties. Almost unheard of, one doctor adds. They begin the medication experiments, trying to find the dosage that will hold him somewhere between flat blackness and euphoric agitation. It takes weeks to get the balance right. During that time, John scales the chain-link fence at the hospital and disappears for a day. He surfaces in the hotel across the river, having a beer in the pub.

I ask about a pass and am amazed to get one the next day. We drive to our old hometown, high in the mountains. As we wind up the steep hill, John talks. "When it began, I took all the knives from the kitchen, I had them all in my arms, and I went upstairs to find her, she was in the bedroom, and I said, Here, you have to put these somewhere, take them away from me, I don't know what I might do. That's how it began."

We find the only bookstore in town, a place with great coffee and armchairs you can sink into. When it's time to head back to the hospital, my brother doesn't resist. He seems more relaxed than I've seen him for a long time. We drive down the long hill, taking the curves we've known since we were children. The enormous discharge pipes of the smelter flash by, painted a cheerful orange.

"Remember when you worked at the smelter?" I ask. "How you used to have to be tested for lead?"

John laughs. "Yeah, when your levels got too high, they moved you to some other part of the smelter."

"What happens to all that lead?"

"Settles in your bones. Never leaves."

We're past the smelter now, driving onto the bridge that flares up over the river in a graceful arc, leading us back to the hospital. I start to laugh. I want to make a joke, a bad one, about John being a human magnet, when I remember that lead doesn't magnetize. I tell him what I was thinking and he laughs. "Well," he says. "I am bipolar."

I glance at my brother, see his face split in his wide grin, and then I'm laughing, laughing so hard I start to cry.

Haunted

LAUREN McGUIRE

When I was a teenager, I had this recurring daydream. As I rode my ten-speed around our suburban subdivision in Worthington, Ohio, I would imagine I was the president of the United States and I would have to choose between my office and offering a stay of execution for my younger brother, who had killed someone. It was an odd vision, as at the time Michael had shown no inclination of being violent or even strange. He was a pretty boy who ran track and was on the gymnastics team. Even though I was student council president, he had more friends than I did.

The dream had no solid basis in reality, nor was it wishful thinking. Each time I dreamt, I would choose saving Michael over having the most powerful job in the world. And yet my waking dream came partially true. More than a dozen years after those days riding my bike around my parents' neighbourhood, my schizophrenic brother killed a drag queen named Gary with a samurai sword.

I remember the phone call from my father the weekend of Michael's arrest. His voice sounded rehearsed as he told me the news.

"Michael is in trouble.

"This time, it is serious.

"He is in jail.

"He stabbed someone.

"And the guy died."

Five sentences, twenty words.

The State of Ohio sought the death penalty. His diagnosis of schizophrenia precluded him from the ultimate punishment, but it was not sufficient for him to be declared not guilty by reason of insanity, which would have allowed him to live in a facility for the mentally ill. He is serving twenty-five years to life in prison.

Now Michael is defined by murder. Everything I think about Michael is in the context of his crime, and every memory has a different hue. It wasn't until after Michael killed Gary that understanding my brother's mind became my mission, my fixation. I couldn't let go of what happened until I understood how this disease could have caused my otherwise peaceful brother to raise a sword against another man.

■　■　■

I remember the first time I thought my brother was crazy. I wonder if others with mentally ill family members have these moments of clarity, the epiphany when they realize their loved one isn't just different or odd but certifiably insane. Four years before his arrest, Michael and I were meeting for lunch at Dalt's in Worthington. It was Christmas 1998, and two months earlier I had a full-term stillbirth, the worst thing that had ever happened to me. I looked around the wood-panelled bar and grill with its brass railings as we waited for a table. I wasn't sure what to expect from this meeting. Part of me was glad to see Michael, but I was also livid he had missed my daughter's funeral, which was attended by more than one hundred of my friends, family, and co-workers. My father had given Michael money to make the trip to Chicago, but he gave it to a friend to bail another friend out of jail.

"Ya know, I thought they were going to pay me back . . ." was his excuse. Not that I needed one—Michael had become increasingly unpredictable and irresponsible. He and I had been close growing up and I needed to talk to him about losing the baby. My seventh grade teacher, Mr. Phillips told my class that siblings are the most important people in our lives: they will know us longer and better than anyone else. They will most likely outlive our parents and we will know them longer than we will know our spouses. I believed Mr. Phillips and viewed Michael in this light. I needed him at Ada's funeral and he had let me down.

I followed Michael as we were led to our table. He had the slow, deliberate walk of an athlete, his shoulders slightly hunched forward from weightlifting. He reminded me of a cheetah: quiet, graceful, and lean, as if he could break into a sprint at any moment. His lithe body could have passed for that of an eighteen-year-old, even though he was twenty-seven.

As we sipped our beers and waited for our quesadillas, Michael said, "Laur, I gotta tell ya something. You are not going to believe it."

He seemed happier and more excited than I had seen him in years. It was as if he just gotten a new puppy. Perhaps he was coming out of his funk, becoming again the brother I had known growing up.

"When I kick the winning goal in the final World Cup Soccer game, I am going to reveal my platform for world peace. You'll see," he said. "It's gonna be awesome."

Platform for world peace rang in my ears. I was perplexed but didn't say anything. I just nodded and went along with the conversation. For the past few years, Michael had talked about playing professional soccer. I had thought of it more as an unattainable dream, but his making the US World Cup team was flat-out delusional. Michael never even played high school soccer. I occasionally imagine I am crossing the finish line at the Olympics when I ride my bike, or have just won Wimbledon after I hit a line drive backhand, but the fantasy ends when the adrenalin stops.

Michael had been talking about playing for the Columbus Crew or some other professional soccer club since he dropped out of the University of Cincinnati, where he had once wanted to study architecture. After floundering at community colleges for a few years, Michael and my father had a heart-to-heart talk. My dad had asked Michael what his life dream and passions were, thinking Michael would choose something practical or follow his childhood dreams of owning a pizza parlour or becoming an architect. He had hoped all Michael needed to get back on track was a good pep talk. My brother's response that he wanted to play professional soccer was the last thing my father expected.

In the previous months, my parents had told me stories of Michael's paranoia. He had refused to leave my father's office until all the other cars left the parking lot, fearing a seventy-year-old lady visiting the dentist across the street was spying on him. Whenever he left the house, Michael had carried his sword over his shoulder in a pool cue case for protection from demons only he knew. I had previously attributed his paranoid behaviour to personality quirks; my parents blamed alcohol and drugs. As the lunch progressed, I realized it was more than that. He talked of world peace in an excited yet practical voice, as if he were telling me he was applying to law school. Michael was lucid and sober: he was nursing a Corona—more water than beer. And there were no darting eyes or incoherent sentences.

Over the course of an hour, Michael changed in my eyes from a brother who was weird, unpredictable, and irresponsible to someone who was insane. Suddenly, I understood everything in Michael's life since he was twenty—from why he couldn't finish college or keep more than fifty dollars in his chequing account, to why the best job he had ever had was running a cash register at a carryout pizza place, to his grandiose ideas about religion. I couldn't be angry with him anymore. *It isn't his fault*, I thought. *He is a bona fide loon.*

My parents had been waiting for him to wake up, grow up, and join the middle class, but it wasn't going to happen. He needed help, and not from therapists who talk to people when they are feeling blue, but from doctors and psychologists who diagnose mental illnesses and could treat him appropriately.

"What is your platform for world peace?" I had asked, stirring my iced tea. I was curious to hear what was running through his mind, to gather information to prove or disprove if he was insane. My gut knew he was crazy, but my rational mind still needed concrete evidence. Being crazy might also not be all bad: the concept of him having a platform of world peace was oddly beautiful and innocent. After having lost a baby, I would have gladly spent my days living in a make-believe world, unattached to reality, floating around in reverie.

"When I kick the winning goal," he said with a beatific smile, "all will be revealed."

I silently nodded because there was nothing I could say to dissuade him from his visions of glory. I felt honoured that he trusted me, that he could tell me what was in the recesses of his soul. Yet his trust began to make me feel responsible: he needed help and he wasn't capable of asking for it himself. Short of telling my parents, I didn't know what to do. I lived more than three hundred miles away in Chicago—there was no way I could participate in any treatment on a day-to-day basis.

I also didn't know much about mental illness. I had thought it was marked by extreme behaviour, like running around in the snow with no clothes on. While Michael was clearly delusional, we could still have a semi-coherent conversation over lunch. It wasn't like he was clucking like a chicken while we were eating.

Finally, when we were driving home after lunch, Michael spoke of Ada.

"Jason's wife had a miscarriage. She was only a few weeks along, and they were really upset. I can't imagine what you went through. I can't. I'm sorry I took up the whole conversation talking about myself." He seemed genuinely sorry, both about Ada and monopolizing the lunch conversation.

"It's okay," I said reassuringly.

"I am really sorry about Ada."

"It's okay." Michael dropped me off at my parents' house and he left without coming inside.

Later that night, I told my dad Michael needed to see someone who could diagnose mental illness. My father told me they had been trying to get Michael to see a psychologist or a psychiatrist, but they couldn't force him to unless he was a danger to himself or others. Michael refused to go—he thought he was fine and that it was the rest of the world that had problems.

■　■　■

After Christmas, I had a dream that I was looking for Michael. I was supposed to meet him on a corner in some sterile, nameless big city. I had just gotten off work and was searching this strange town in a suit and heels trying to find him. I was checking my watch when I saw my parents coming out of a subway station in the middle of a crowd. I asked them where Michael was, and my dad touched Michael's elbow. He was unrecognizable. He was stooped over, a few inches shorter than my father. Michael looked like he did when he was fourteen—the same height and skinny, skinny, skinny— except he had a vacant stare and was holding an empty paper cup like the street people who asked for spare change on the corner near my apartment. It dawned on me Michael had had a lobotomy; I was jolted awake. I'd rather have Michael be a little off-centre than not have him at all.

Now, I look back at that lunch at Dalt's and see our lives slowly falling forward. I am most disappointed with what I didn't do with my sense that my brother was crazy. I sat on it. I was busy with my own life. I thought his insanity was interesting and curious. It never occurred to me that it could be dangerous. If anything, I felt at ease knowing Michael's erratic behaviour wasn't his fault.

I wish I had done more for Michael after our conversation at Dalt's, but it wasn't in me at the time. I had enough turmoil in my own life after losing Ada. I was still grieving and didn't have the energy to deal with Michael's problems, which seemed minor compared to mine. I couldn't think of anything other than wanting children. I knew my next pregnancy would be an emotional roller coaster: I would be excited to be pregnant again but terrified that I might lose another baby. Plus I carried the family responsibility to have kids, as Michael clearly was not headed in that direction.

The reality of Michael's illness was far from the romantic images I'd had after our lunch at Dalt's. Two years later, my parents were desperate. Michael's paranoia had become debilitating and caring for him was beyond their capabilities. They talked to psychologists and psychiatrists to get Michael into inpatient treatment. At all turns, my parents were thwarted. Regardless of what any of the health-care professionals said or how delusional and dysfunctional Michael had become, he couldn't receive involuntary treatment in Ohio unless he was a danger to himself or others.

Two years after our lunch at Dalt's, I brought my six-month-old daughter to Columbus to visit my parents and Michael for Christmas. My mother, the baby, and I went to lunch at da Vinci's, where Michael was bussing tables. He refused to stop by our table, so I put my baby on my hip and went to the back hall to find him.

"Why don't you stop by the house?" I asked him.

"Mom and Dad don't want me there," Michael said. My mother and Michael fought so often, I stopped asking my parents about the latest row.

"What's going on?" I asked, assuming it was the same old story of him not working enough or smoking pot.

"You won't believe this," Michael told me. "Dad tried to shove me down the stairs. He started yelling and shoving and I left."

I was appalled. Usually my father was the stable one, the one who didn't engage Michael in arguments or scream at him over his lifestyle choices—that was my mother's domain. I normally stood in the middle, thinking my parents were too hard on Michael but still understanding their angst about their son.

When I had my father alone, I asked him about it. He was unusually defensive.

"You don't understand," he said. "I was trying to get him to hit me. If he hit me, we could have sent him to NetCare to get evaluated. They would have checked him in for three days and he could have been diagnosed."

■ ■ ■

Two weeks after Michael's arrest for killing Gary, the social workers at the jail realized Michael was not responding as someone arrested for a violent crime usually acts. My mother called Michael's assigned social worker and told her Michael's history of erratic behaviour. He was promptly moved to the jail's psych floor. Six months later, Michael was moved to a mental health facility, where he was diagnosed with schizophrenia. He refused to participate in his own defence, and for three years was declared incompetent to stand trial. Eventually, he was medicated against his will and brought to trial in August 2005.

The trial was a local media circus. The four television channels in Columbus, Ohio, covered the case. Against the advice of his attorneys, Michael took the stand. When asked by the prosecution if he knew it was wrong to kill people, he said yes. "I pray everyday for God to forgive me." Despite the fact that Michael was deemed schizophrenic by every psychologist and psychiatrist who met him, and despite the fact that Michael was convinced Gary and his friends killed Michael's friend Craig and were then going to kill him, Michael failed to be declared not guilty by reason of insanity. He said he knew the difference between right and wrong, the minimum standard for sanity in Ohio.

■ ■ ■

Almost two years after his trial, I finally had the courage to attend a class sponsored by the National Alliance for the Mentally Ill (NAMI). Michael had been diagnosed with schizophrenia, but I didn't understand it. I knew he was delusional, paranoid, and generally odd, but I didn't understand how they connected together and ruined his life. It was as if schizophrenia was a foreign idiom: I knew the literal meaning but had no context to understand the wider impacts of the disease.

At the NAMI classes, I learned that the three main side effects of a major mental illness are the inability to hold a job, to live independently, and to maintain significant relationships. With that information, the story of Michael's life crystallized. Before he killed his friend, Michael's life was chaos for nearly a decade. Rarely could he hold a busboy job longer than six weeks, and he relied on my parents and his wide network of friends for food and shelter. He'd couch surf at one person's house for a few days before moving on to the next, only to circle back a few weeks or months later. Michael's peculiarities, strange habits, and general dysfunction now fit into a pattern.

Now that his basic needs are taken care of by the State of Ohio, the side effects of his illness are gone. He has a place to sleep every night and he gets three meals a day. His prison jobs—tidying the gym for an hour a day and occasionally filling in for the yoga teacher—are more like hobbies than an occupation. While he doesn't have a significant other, his relationship with my parents is far more congenial than it was before his arrest. He is more stable but far from cured.

In the summer of 2009, my husband, John, and I flew in from Seattle to visit my brother in prison. The Chillicothe Correctional Institution is the fourth prison he has been assigned to since his trial. Since I only see him once a year, it took me a while to absorb the changes in his face and learn the new cadence of his voice. This time, his face seemed even more lined, his jaw more chiselled. His voice had a southern Ohio drawl. Within twenty minutes of our visit, Michael's voice morphed back into his old crisp Midwestern accent, complete with proper grammar.

Michael came in and talked about problems with his bowels, a persistent fixation with complaints and symptoms for which the prison physicians could find no medical explanation. Michael had quit the church choir because he couldn't last the hour-long practice without needing to use the restroom several times. John is a physician, so Michael peppered him with questions about his upcoming colonoscopy and hernia surgery.

The three of us played Super-Mega Scrabble, where we used two bags of tiles on one board. Michael had memorized the two-letter word list I had mailed him last year. I didn't talk much while we were playing. It was difficult to carry on a conversation while trying to figure out what word I could spell with three Os, two Is, an E, and an R.

When John and I came back from lunch, we put the game aside and Michael talked about prison life.

"I don't know why these guys have to act so tough," Michael said. "What is the point?"

Like our conversation at Dalt's years ago, I nodded without comment, but this time Michael was the rational one living in an irrational world. *He doesn't get it*, I thought. *He doesn't understand the prison mentality and he doesn't belong here.*

Overall the visit was pleasant. Too pleasant, in fact. I was slightly unsettled by how easy it was to spend time with him. The lines of my memory were blurring, and it seemed as if the past dozen years had never happened. Perhaps the murder and trial were imagined, a delusion of my own. It was as if the Michael I knew growing up had died in his early twenties, and now I was sitting here with the ghost of the boy I used to know. But he wasn't a ghost, he was a man anchored to an act committed years ago during a period of severe psychosis.

After the visit, I had a most disturbing thought.

"I think killing someone and landing in prison saved Michael's life," I told John as we walked through the prison parking lot. "And that horrifies me. I imagine he would be dead by now living on the streets."

"Why couldn't he have been treated before he killed Gary, which would have saved two lives?" I said. I was back to where I was seven years earlier, asking the same question. I also thought about where we might have been had Michael not been arrested or died on the streets. I doubt John and I would sit down with him for hours listening to his philosophy. He most likely would have been talking about his latest row with my parents, or how the world was trying to screw him by not giving him his chance to play professional soccer.

Here it is: Michael is stable, and the rest of the world had to suffer for that to happen. The ripple of his illness was great. On one shore, Gary was killed and his friends and family mourned his death. On the other, my family suffered, knowing someone we love took someone's life. My father seems to have resigned himself with my brother's fate. When I asked him how he copes, he told me, "I've never gotten over it. I've just gotten used to it."

I would think about my brother the first thing in the morning and the last thing before I fell asleep every day for seven years after his arrest. Slowly, other parts of my life—mainly my own children—reclaimed those dark places in my heart and brought me light. And yet I am perplexed when I look back at those moments that foreshadowed Michael's downfall. Of course, there were moments when he was clearly detached from reality. But it is the quiet moments, the ones on the cusp, that make me ponder. Those moments where I look back and see the course of Michael's life turning, slowly changing from where I imagined it would have gone. Those moments didn't come with trumpets heralding disaster. They were quiet, like a teenaged girl's daydream on a bike.

Pennies in My Pocket
Stories of My Brother
LAURA TRUNKEY

Months after his twentieth birthday, my brother lay on our mother's front lawn, certain he was dying. He was home alone but for the cat, who likely skimmed against his legs before stalking toward the fence and the promise of robins.

Perhaps my brother had wanted to go farther than the lawn: down the driveway, up the street, away. But he only made it to the garden; he lay near tall stalks of foxgloves that leaned sideways, too heavy for their stems, and closed his eyes.

Neighbourhood boys passed on their way to the basketball courts, their balls beating a steady pulse against the sidewalk. The boys didn't notice my brother behind the oak trees in the yard. Or did but only saw a young man asleep on the grass, pale skin flushed pink, arms outstretched. If they looked closely they would have seen he was already unravelling: his clothes were dirty, stiff with his smell. His bleached hair was tangled and his fingernails untrimmèd.

Did my brother hear the basketballs, the snatches of gúitar riffs and pounding bass that slipped from unrolled windows of passing cars? Did he hear the bell on the cat's collar, as it stepped over his legs to drink from the tin beneath the water faucet in our mother's garden?

I imagine these sounds were imperceptible to him. He heard none of them, nor did he feel last autumn's acorns beneath him, small marbles the lawnmower passed over. As he waited for our mother to return, his entire world dissolved. All that was left was the shiver of sparking electricity in his chest.

My brother didn't know what would follow: the neighbour sitting behind him in our mother's car, holding his hands from the door handle, nineteen hours in the Emergency Room, a string of intakes at the Pavilion, the mental health ward, assessment after assessment, and finally a diagnosis: schizophrenia. A word that has the power to procure bottles of pills, government money, caseworkers with action plans and recovery goals, but can also shatter worlds: whispered friend to friend, a game of broken telephone until the phone's no longer ringing.

This story, my brother on the lawn alone, is one I can't help telling myself. It snags other thoughts, other memories so that I summon it without meaning to. And I'm no longer sure what's true and what's imagined: are the cat, the child witnesses, the foxgloves all invented? It's not the event I remember but the stories I was told; I wasn't there.

■ ■ ■

Because it's genetic.

When it comes to gene pools, ours is muddied with mental illness. My father's mother married a good Mormon man, birthed two children in Albuquerque, where the mountains are pink as watermelon, and when things went sour she moved to another city, married another man—less good—and gave him four gifts: two girls and two boys. She raised these six children in a place where they could leave home running and reach, in one direction, the Las Vegas strip and, in the other, the Nevada Desert. She raised them while working behind the till in a convenience store, she raised them when she was depressed, when she was manic, when she was with lithium and without. And when her husband was dead and her six children gone, she called them on the telephone. She called at 3:00 AM and said her postal code was 90210. She called and asked her grandchildren, *How old are you now?* Every time, the same question. *How old are you? How old are you?* She sent paper doilies with our names scrawled on them for Christmas presents.

Why is she like that? I wanted to know. My father said some people just turned out that way.

■ ■ ■

Because I feared it into being.

By first grade, the year my parents divorced, I was afraid of everything from elevators to wiener dogs. I had stomachaches not detected by ultrasounds or cured by prescriptions for chalky liquids. *Nervous stomachaches*, my gran said. *Like your mother.*

Most of all, I was afraid that something would happen to my brother.

I had nightmares about it: that he stuck his finger in a light socket, choked on the Halloween candy hidden in his dresser, was murdered by my cousin during a violent game of tag. I had daymares too—a sixth sense about his well-being that was generally inauspicious and incorrect. It would strike me while playing with friends up the street, while in the shower, while reading comic books on my bedroom floor. I would run immediately to find him, and then I'd hover over him until I was convinced he was not faking ordinariness; he was actually okay.

If James were well, chances are these daymares would be forgotten, but now that he's been diagnosed I still have that sixth sense. It's honed to his illness, and it's much more accurate than before. When the pauses in his sentences stretch, when he stops wearing his glasses, when he wants to sell everything he owns and buy back everything he has ever sold, when his eyes are dull and his expression is flat and he can't tell a joke even when it's easy, even when the punchline is on a platter in front of him, I know James is having symptoms: hallucinations, delusions. And I want to hover still.

■ ■ ■

Because it's biological.

Years before James lay in the front yard expecting death, our mother placed him on the lawn of the neighbour's house while he seized and then stopped breathing. She bent over her only son as cars passed, as cars passed, as cars passed. James had grand mal seizures as a child, perhaps the result of being born with a skull fracture. Fevers could precipitate them and so could head injuries; he wore a white hockey helmet at soccer practice, during gym class, and while playing in the yard with friends.

I was rarely around for James's seizures, but the stories of them (told by my mother, by my gran when she arrived at school to take me for the "sleepovers" that only ever had one cause) were like the pennies my granddad and I collected on walks: the longer I held on to them, the more polished they became, the more deeply they were etched in my memory.

There is an evening of my childhood I remember clearly; I am eight and James is four. My brother has a fever, and Mum runs cool water in the bathtub and places him inside. He sits still and silent, and this is proof that he is sick. Our mother has always said she can tell when I'm unwell because I'm irritable, mean, the worst version of myself. My brother is the opposite: he suffers silently. Every couple of minutes our mother places the metal tip of the thermometer under my brother's armpit. She recites the numbers into the telephone, which is pinned against her ear with her shoulder. When she finally towels James off and lays him on her bed, the pullout couch in the living room, I know what will happen before the seizing starts. I slip from the house into the side yard, where I hide beneath branches of the oak tree, waiting for him to be cured.

■ ■ ■

Because of what he eats.

My brother's epilepsy ended with the elimination of cow's milk from his diet and a Ziploc bag full of vitamins from an orthomolecular psychiatrist (horse pills and foul-smelling liquid that lingered on his breath and stained any surface it touched iodine-brown). Eventually even James's helmet and medical alert bracelet disappeared.

James has not had a seizure since he was a child, but he drinks milk again. Helping him with his eighth move in three years I avoid the living room, where hundreds of bought, gifted, and scavenged records loom over dirty socks and food-encrusted dishes. Instead I go to the refrigerator. I pull out a half-empty four-litre jug of milk, and place it in the laundry hamper beside me. The hamper has already carted the contents of James's bedroom dresser to his new apartment, as well as his extensive Kraft dinner and Chef Boyardee collections.

"How can you ever expect to feel better if you eat this crap?" I say. "You're allergic to dairy products."

He's taking pudding cups from the cupboard above the stove and transferring them to a box on the counter, and he doesn't turn around. "I'm fine."

"Two litres of Coke." I pull the bottle from the otherwise empty vegetable crisper and hold it up for James to see.

"Diet Coke," he says. "It's for losing weight." Three years ago when James was well, this kind of statement, delivered deadpan, would have been his idea of a joke. But I can tell he's serious. James's weight has almost doubled since he was diagnosed, a combination of the medication and his diet. He's worried about it.

"The fact that something says diet on the label doesn't mean it makes you lose weight."

He just stares at me.

"If you want to lose weight, you should drink water, not pop. And you should exercise. You should . . ." But I stop the spiel when I notice the box on the counter, now completely full of pudding cups. There are still more in the cupboard above his head.

"How many fucking pudding cups does one person need?" It is impossible to be rational under these circumstances.

■ ■ ■

Because I didn't protect him.

At home and at school, once he was old enough to attend, my brother and I played together only when I'd have him, only when his presence was necessary. I wrote songs and trained James to sing them into our mother's tape recorder, creating permanent records of James's pre–speech therapy voice. He was an eager pupil, and my lessons extended beyond music. I dressed him in leotards for rhythmic gymnastics instruction in the living room and I taught him to build forts. We used bedsheets and couch cushions to make elaborate caves from the dining room furniture, spaces only we were small enough to enter. James thought when people couldn't see him he was invisible; he wore dark sunglasses to the doctor's office and kept a dome tent erected in his bedroom until he was eight or nine. Our sheet-caves had similar appeal. We lay side by side in silence.

Mostly, though, I chose to be alone with my collections (eggshells, bird's nests, beach glass, stones), and James played with his cookie tin of crayons and his "good beat" music, a mix-tape made for him by my mother's friend, which he listened to daily while performing high kicks in a karate uniform, the belt tied around his head. We existed on separate planes.

■ ■ ■

Because no one noticed sooner.

By the time James turned nineteen it was obvious to everyone that something was wrong. The boy who hurdled his way to the BC championships, spent hours at the piano playing ragtime tunes without being cajoled into practising, wallpapered my mother's living room with oil paintings, had a series of invitations to choose from every weekend, suddenly became a young man who wouldn't go to college classes, wouldn't take phone calls, and wouldn't shower. He yelled at our mother, threatened her enough that she hid the knives and matches and carted the photo albums to a friend's house. James spent all his time in his bedroom, and all that time was spent doing one thing: reorganizing and rearranging everything he owned.

My brother always ordered his possessions. As a child, he lined up his toys by size, his records by colour. When our mother collected strewn clothes and toys from the living room and kitchen, and refused to give them back until bedrooms were cleaned, she meant my bedroom only. I was the one who dumped every dresser drawer on the floor with the intent to clean my room, and cried once I saw the mess, claiming I had no place to put *anything*. I hid things under beds and stuffed them in closets. But my brother's world always made sense, was always pristine.

This reordering was different, though: frantic, obsessive. He moved his bed around his room, yet no matter where he placed it he never seemed to sleep. Our mum compiled notes for the doctor. She gave me lists of things to talk to James about when I called from Halifax, where I was working in a shelter for homeless youth. But whenever anyone asked my brother how he was, he said only one word: *fine*.

I flew home to visit when his first year of art school was almost over; everything had changed. When James and I both lived at home, even when he couldn't eat dairy and I wouldn't eat meat, my mother made family dinners every night. This was the time we spent together. Perfect fork handling was expected, and there was candlelight sometimes, but this was so my brother, a skilled food dissector, couldn't see well enough to separate the vegetables from the rest of his meal. These dinners weren't the civilized sort that I encountered at friends' houses. There was no talk of current events, no *What did you learn at school?* Instead, there was my brother's comedy routine: James snorting juice out his nose and tipping off his chair onto the floor, me running to the hallway holding my stomach and screaming: *stop making me laugh*.

During my visit, dinners were silent. James stayed in his room most of the time, drawing in a sketchbook that contained nothing but heavily inked scribbles, claws and teeth visible at the edges of each page. When he finally agreed to a game of cards, he stared past me at the wall and twisted his neck in circles, grinning at nothing. I talked him through each move until I snapped.

In Halifax, half the boys on my caseload had mental illnesses and I should have been able to see the signs. But James was my brother—he was different. I followed him into his room and demanded he tell me what was wrong, why was he acting the way he was, did he realize how worried people were about him? He punched me, he swore, he cried—but he admitted to nothing. When he did confess to hearing voices, it was to a friend. This friend told his mother, who told ours. A week later James was referred to a psychiatrist by our family doctor. He was put on an antipsychotic drug and on the waiting list for a psychiatric assessment at the hospital. But the list was long, the psychiatrist told my mother. It could be months before they admitted him for testing. The fastest way in was through Emergency.

■ ■ ■

Because I wasn't there.

I was back in Halifax when James was admitted to hospital. He took the Dexedrine our family doctor prescribed combined with Risperdal prescribed by the psychiatrist, and then he called our mother's cell to say he was having a heart attack. She arrived home to find him lying on the lawn in her side yard, shaking. It took her and the man in the duplex's upstairs unit to get him into the car, James trying to throw the doors open and jump onto the road. Once in Emergency, James bolted and had to be chased and dragged back. The triage nurse confiscated his Dexedrine, said the two drugs should never be taken at once.

This first trip to Emergency, my brother waited for nineteen hours with our mother beside him. He chose to sit in the silence of the padded room at the end of the hall rather than on a stretcher in the corridor. The next morning, just before noon, he was given a bed at the Pavilion. Hospital security escorted James to the concrete building on the other side of the grounds. Our mother was told that if she drove him home to pack it would be the equivalent of "checking out" and he'd lose his bed.

James remained in the hospital past his first and then his second estimated release date. Some of his tests were inconclusive. At first, no one was sure exactly how to label his illness.

Our mother was allowed to visit with him in the afternoons. She could take him for coffee at the Starbucks across the street from the hospital; she was not supposed to take him home. But often she did: he wouldn't use the shower on the ward, wouldn't eat. When he went into the dining room, he said, he made people choke. His roommate told him he could read his mind, then stole his headphones and wore them around the ward.

When I called, the nurses transferred me to the phone in the hallway; usually, though, James didn't answer the page. I started looking for him in the boys on my caseload. There was the one who medicated himself with alcohol, who we discharged time after time because he didn't return to claim his bed. Instead he ended up in the drunk tank or passed out someplace outside: a park, an empty lot, the graveyard down the street. There was the boy who was terrified of getting out of bed, and the boy whose walls talked when he was in his room at night. None of these boys were my brother, though sometimes I caught glimpses of him in them. I carried their stories around with me, let them keep me awake at night and push away other thoughts during the day. I felt I must help these boys, all these boys.

I moved back to Victoria.

■   ■   ■

What do our memories say about us? My father remembered his mother as the woman who made everything hard. I started writing her when it was too late; she had a stroke the day after I put the letter in the mail. But a childhood friend of my father's read my letter to her on a visit, and then wrote to tell me why he still made the drive from LA to Las Vegas twice a month to see her. To him, she was the woman who ran the only convenience store in town a black man could enter and get a smile along with his change. An adult who saw possibility in every kid's hoop dream.

I've heard it said when you remember something it's not the facts you recall, but your last examination of that memory. That though they may seem fixed, memories are stories that shift with each telling. Did my father's friend see my grandmother's illness, or had he looked beyond this detail so many times that in his stories it had no place? Did my father recall his mother's resilience, or had "crazy" bulldozed everything beautiful that grew around it, despite it? Though both of these versions must contain truth, my father and his friend chose different stories, different pennies to hold on to.

The pennies that tell my truths about James, the ones I can't let go of, are the times he was fragile, in danger, and I was powerless to help: the lawn stories. But what if I picked another coin to polish?

If I could empty my pockets and start fresh, I would say that when I was seven I filled a bag with underwear and my stuffed rabbit and set off to find another family and that my brother, only three and unable to recognize my bravado for what it was, chased me down the street. With the first glance over my shoulder, I knew I couldn't leave. My brother was pumping his arms and gaining ground. I would say that this story, in which I pick him up and carry him to the grass by the oak tree in our front yard, snot smearing my shoulder, fingers digging into my neck, is the only lawn story worth remembering.

I would say that my brother never fell—not swiftly, not thoroughly, not at all. That he only stumbled. And that while falling signals an end to a story, stumbling is only an interruption.

Only Love Taps

NICOLE MELCHIONDA

When I was thirteen, my brother tried to dismember his arm with a kitchen knife. I came home from school to an unusually empty house and found the weapon lying on the kitchen table. I later learned that he was taken to a psychiatric hospital in an ambulance, because he claimed he had a microchip implanted in him and that his family wasn't *really* his family. I didn't dare visit him. When my parents left me alone in our vast four-bedroom home, I held that same knife to my wrist for a long time, fantasizing about my suicide.

I couldn't cut. I've never cut myself beyond the use of thumbtacks, a method my friend taught me when I was twelve because the marks usually faded by the next day and it rarely drew blood. My brother spent years moulding me into a self-loathing anti-human, but no matter how hard he pushed me to kill myself, I couldn't give in to what I believed was our joint desire for suicide. Somebody would have to find my body, and that fact alone is what kept me alive.

I developed an alter ego to conceal my depression. I often think about a picture of me smiling sleepily at a swim meet when, just the night before, Ryan violently shook me awake, dragged me out of bed so forcefully that my body thudded against the hardwood floor, and then beat me because I refused to tell him the password to the family computer he kept damaging with viruses. No one that day suspected I was mentally ebbing, because I always performed at my best, as an athlete and a human. No one really knew who I was. My mother met my true self once she forced me to visit a doctor after she grew tired of my excessive absences from school. I begged her not to take me, promising I wouldn't miss any more classes, but she was afraid of the stranger I was becoming. I was afraid too, but for different reasons. I didn't want to face anyone who had the power to diagnose me and force my illness into the open where I could become even more ostracized. I already knew what I was harboring inside me. I didn't want some white coat pitying me.

But when the doctor asked me why I'd come to his office, I told him that I was depressed. My mother's face tightened. Her arms folded. The doctor sighed and the ticking of his office clock reverberated through every cell in my body. The smiling zoo animals painted on all four walls started laughing, staring right through me, closing in on me to better examine the real exhibit. I felt myself leaving my body to escape that room.

"What are your symptoms?"

"I can't get out of bed, I have no appetite, I am no longer interested in things that used to interest me, I am sad, and when I'm not sad I feel nothing at all." I provided the laundry list of symptoms I researched on Google before the appointment to make sure there would be no confusion or any reason to bring me back to the doctor ever again.

"Have you felt suicidal?"

All the time.

"No, never."

I was not going to be strapped to a hospital bed on suicide watch.

I performed my duties as a circus monkey and was rewarded with a fast diagnosis. A two-minute conversation was enough to determine that I was mentally unfit to take care of myself. He suggested a therapist and the possibility of medication, but I refused both. To this day, I choose not to see a therapist, partially out of pride, and I reject any prescriptions because I've never put anything in my body that could fuck me up even more. I don't know if I inherited the depression from somewhere in my genes, but I always attributed my stubbornness to my father.

When I'd started getting depressed, I took advantage of my mother's trust and lied that I was sick. One time, when I missed around a week of school, she assumed I just didn't want to do any work. I shoved my fingers down my throat and showed her my vomit just to avoid any human interaction, because when I wasn't alone, I was no longer myself. To this day, I still carry on with my ritualistic smile and I show enthusiasm for everything, because I've realized how tiring it is to answer the same questions every day about whether or not I am okay. Most people's first impression of me is that I'm ditzy, but that's okay because that judgment usually deters them from really getting to know me.

It's not that I don't want to talk to anyone, it's that no one can fix me. Even if I did see a therapist like my mom still begs me to do, I know that they cannot open my skull and fix the broken synapses, that although this disease doesn't have to be terminal, I will always be a carrier. Only as I write this essay do I realize how painfully honest the lies to my mother really were, and how my absences from school were, perhaps, necessary.

When I was younger, I was a lot less sympathetic toward Ryan and the addictions he had in his desperate attempts to self-medicate. I thought he was weak and that he didn't care about how his actions impacted us. My biggest regret was when I was around fourteen and told Ryan that I wished he would kill himself so our family could get better and heal. Yes, his drug-induced states had wreaked havoc on our once close-knit family that endures to this day, but did I have to be so cruel as to tell another human being to die? In that moment, I became my brother, and he became me.

"I've already tried three times," he said back then as he burst into tears, something he'd never done in front of me before.

I cried too, which was an all-too-common occurrence for me at that time, and I held him tightly to bind him to the earth. I hated him and loved him and wished he was never born and wanted to save him all while hating myself. My arms clung to him with rage and adoration as we sobbed about how irreversibly fucked up our lives would be so long as we each lived.

I was too young to understand when Ryan was himself and when he was high on all kinds of drugs. He abused me for around ten years of my childhood and adolescence and, when he was high, he never remembered what he'd done to me. One night, while I was sitting on the couch and my parents had gone to bed, he sauntered into the room and plopped down next to me with an almost empty bottle of wine in hand. He had drunk that whole bottle, but was barely even buzzed. Even though I was the sober one, I can only recall fragments of the conversation that ensued. I told him that his assaults left bruises on my body.

His glazed eyes spilled alcoholic tears, perhaps pure vodka, and the television cast haunting blue shadows upon his face, making him look cadaverous. "I never meant to hurt you. Those were only love taps," he said.

I choked on my tears and considered how sick I must be for wishing that all those years of abuse had been purely physical. I would've easily traded each cruel remark for a broken bone instead because I knew my body was more resilient than my mind could ever be.

The reason why it took me ten years to own my disease is because when I actually did ask for help, I was rejected. One day in my high school freshman year, I cautiously sat down with someone who I thought was my best friend. I'd known her since preschool. She was the first friend I'd ever made, and we grew up like sisters.

I managed to gurgle out that I had depression. She cocked her head in polite consideration for a brief moment, beamed radiantly, and chirped, "Just go on medication." She got up and left me sitting alone. That was all she ever had to say to me about that subject, like most other things those days.

I tried vaporizing my sickness every way I knew how. I kept busy, I took up many hobbies, I ate well, and I exercised rigorously. When I was twelve, I almost instantly morphed from the chubby kid who ate her feelings into a svelte, curvaceous woman who received compliments on her six-pack whenever friends snuck peeks in the changing room. I swam six days a week for three hours each day, never missing a practice, selfishly showing up with plagues of flus, colds, and other highly transmittable illnesses. I became obsessed and, with a year's work, I went from being in horrible shape to the number one backstroker in New Hampshire and an invitee to swim at meets held at Harvard and in Europe. I used swimming as an escape from my brother, and all the times I wanted to throw up from overexertion made me think about the physical, verbal, and mental abuse that was waiting for me at home.

It came as no surprise that I burned out. I slowly tapered off my swimming career and gained forty pounds in the year after I stopped. My brother told me I was fat, worthless, and unlovable, so that's what I became. In an attempt to gain control of my life again, I developed an eating disorder. Sometimes I would "fast" for days, sometimes I would binge, sometimes I would violate my throat with my hands until bile came up. Some days I wouldn't leave bed, some days I would not allow myself to eat or do anything pleasurable until I ran ten miles. I maintained this lifestyle for all four years of high school before I left for college at age seventeen. In my college dorm, I knew I would no longer have the luxury to hide behind locked doors while I did my dirty deeds. I was sick of being sick, tired of being tired, and fed up with being fat. I started treating myself with kindness and, sure enough, the weight began to drop off. I slowly realized that, if I genuinely took care of myself,

I'd be happier and healthier, even if the depression would always tear at my gray matter.

When I was twelve, I started writing in order to combat loneliness. In one poem, when I embarrassingly believed every poem needed to rhyme and each new line had to be capitalized, I explained my compulsion:

> I write to express my sorrow
> All the emotions left unsaid
> I write because my paper listens
> When no one else did

As simplistic as that stanza may be, I still feel it burn beneath my sternum. My brother and all the hardships that have manifested in my life from the hate-spawn he birthed inside me have created the most frustrating contradiction. I write to intimately dissect myself, but each time I approach my brother lyrically, I spew shit. Poems become forced and cliché, and nothing I write ever begins to encapsulate the complex thoughts and emotions I have, so there's this huge, essential part of myself that's forcibly untapped because I'm overcome with ambivalence. No one is one-dimensional, so although it would be easier to pen Ryan as the villain, I've seen his beautiful, selfless parts, too. In some ways, I feel as if I functioned without a *corpus callosum* during my adolescence. One hemisphere of my brain operated with the belief that Ryan was good, while the other half loathed his existence and saw him as a monster. Whichever side had control that day dictated whether I loved or hated Ryan, with no in-between. I knew how illogical and unhealthy this was, which is why I tried to use my poetry as a bridge to connect the two hemispheres, but I never could write something that satisfied both halves of my brain. I have deserted hundreds of half-finished poems about a man who never cares to ask my parents how my life turned out when he calls them, yet I still can't help but wonder if he misses me or if he's sorry.

My mother chastises me for severing all ties with him, and sometimes I hate her. *He's your brother. He's your family. My sister gave me a black eye once. It's what children do. You have to talk to him at some point. You have to learn how to forgive. I think you're making this into a bigger deal than it was. He didn't sexually abuse you, did he?* But what she doesn't understand is that I think I have forgiven him, even if he's marred my skin with remnants of his abuse and degenerated my brain with reptilian reflexes. I no longer harbor resentment toward my parents for what happened, because I know how he abused them as well, how many of my mother's tears were hidden behind her bedroom door, how my parents did everything they could to quell the unquellable. No matter how many times Ryan got arrested, no matter how many expensive therapists my parents took him to, no matter how much love and patience they gave him, he didn't want to better himself.

Any time I face my body dysmorphia in the mirror, I ask myself whose voice I'm really hearing and I'm able to shake away the illusion most of the time. Though my muscles no longer ache with anger, the many years I've spent slowly chiseling away my hatred have left behind a residue of sadness and frustration I can't ignore.

I know my mother loves me. She loves all of her children equally, and perhaps that's what troubles me most. My father does not tolerate Ryan's self-induced crises, but my mother is an enabler and refuses to listen to me when I try to reason with her. She prioritizes his needs over her other three children's, but I also realize that since we are not so problematic, she doesn't have to baby us. When she refuses to love her child any less despite all of the incriminating evidence I have on my side, I remind myself that no decent person would shame someone for quitting cigarettes or alcohol, so I don't allow my mother's criticisms to guilt me into relapse just because my toxin happens to be familial. Accepting the extent of the damage he's done to our family would probably be a burden that would end her. All she wants is to have a

Christmas where everyone in the family can handle being under the same roof.

Despite the occasional whirls of encumbering grief that strike me late at night when I try to sleep, I am okay now—really okay, not the okay I would I say when everything was wrong but I wanted to be left alone. Of course I still have depression and anxiety, but I no longer let my life be defined by my illness. I no longer wish to die. I've found coping mechanisms powerful enough to make me forget a large percentage of the time that I am afflicted. I have to accredit most of my solidity to my boyfriend and antidote, George, who has stayed with me for three years while I deal with my insecurities, guilt, jealousy, panic attacks, and crippling anxiety that plagued the beginning of our relationship. He holds my hand when we go to the grocery store, since going alone is a terrifying feat. He cradles me like a child when my lungs compress and sputter for air as my heart palpitates and I believe I'm actually dying. George is the only person I've allowed myself to be vulnerable with, the only person who has known and loved and cared for my body, the only person who has made me feel accepted, worthy, human. He taught me how to view myself through his eyes and not Ryan's, and now my panic attacks are few and far between. For the first time in my life, I am strong and know that I will remain so.

Habits become instinct, though, when they've had a decade to become practiced and learned. Around six months into the relationship, I mistook George for a fraction of a second for Ryan. He raised his hand mid-stretch and I cringed, because I feared that he was going to beat my skull.

Some things cannot be left behind.

Perhaps Ryan would be surprised to know I still keep a collage of our childhood photos hanging on my bedroom wall, but only of ones when I am no older than three. When I look at the cute, chubby, mystified-by-everything baby that I was, I feel sorry for all she doesn't know is coming, that the little boy with skinny legs next to her in so many of my early photos will obliterate everything she once thought was good about the world.

I've distanced myself so much from that little girl that it feels like she's not me, that I was born at eighteen. Sometimes I feel her loss as my own, but I have and always will treasure what she learned through her grief. Although she and I always possessed the strength to rip ourselves to shreds, we've learned we're stronger when we don't.

Times Long Past

Covering for My Father

DOUGLAS TODD

My first memory of my father is visiting him behind bars. The wide door at the end of the long hall was made of steel, painted white. It was thicker than my little fist. To open the door, the warden raised a long metal handle and pushed it sideways, as if he were providing entry to a cattle barn.

Inside the large, gloomy room in Essondale mental hospital in the Vancouver suburb of Coquitlam, I saw that the grimy windows had bars. About two dozen people sat still in smoke-filled haze. Most were staring, hunched over. Out of it.

I was four years old and my mother and older brother and I were visiting my dad, Harold. He was kept inside a high-security ward at Essondale, which was later to be called Riverview Mental Hospital. My dad shuffled meekly over to us, and the wardens allowed us to take him out for three hours on a Sunday drive in my mother's black Ford, which had running boards. It was the late 1950s. Not a good time to have schizophrenia.

Why my dad was locked up was beyond me. I knew he was seriously sick. But he seemed completely passive, about as threatening as the red-breasted robins that fed in the cherry tree in the backyard of our East Vancouver home. Maybe the bars were there to stop the inmates from jumping out the fourth-storey windows to a merciful death. My young brain could see the reasoning.

Sunday drives with my dad became an almost weekly routine. We'd motor around, visit a park, throw rocks into a lake, go for ice cream or lunch. My dad spoke in monosyllables, if at all. The expression "painfully boring" could have been created for these dutiful events.

I guess my mother, Mary, brother, Dave, and I went on the regular visits because my dad seemed to appreciate them. We could tell at the end by the way he smiled wanly, waving goodbye with a floppy hand.

I found out later my mom's mom didn't think it was a good idea for my brother and I to go on these visits. But my dad's parents believed it was the moral thing to do. I still don't know who was right. But I do know my mom, brother, and I always tried to be as cheerful as we could; no one ever complained.

After a few years of these Sunday visits, it was time for me to head off to school. I joined my neighbourhood friends in walking to grade one at Sir Richard McBride Elementary School in East Vancouver.

That's when I first heard the put-down "mental." A kid hurled the epithet across the gravel schoolyard at someone. It hit home at that moment that whatever it was that was happening to my dad was not only horrible, it was something for which I should also feel ashamed.

This produced silence. But I didn't consciously realize I was keeping a secret until we had moved to North Vancouver and I was thirteen. That's when my best friend, in talking to my mother, referred to my uncle, George, who shared our home with us, as my father.

I guess I had wanted it to look to my new friends like I was in a normal family. But my mom said I had to tell the truth.

■   ■   ■

Just around the time I was born, my dad, who my mom always describes as "a nice man," apparently started acting strangely.

Harold had been an ambulance driver in France in the Second World War, had many friends (who called him "Harry"), was a good athlete, and had completed a commerce degree at the University of BC. But he apparently hadn't been working effectively as an actuary at several forestry companies. Despite not being an executive at the MacMillan-Bloedel lumber company, for instance, he was insisting on using the executive washroom. He was fired.

His parents wouldn't initially believe anything was seriously wrong with him, suggesting my mother was just being critical and unsupportive. My mother, meanwhile, was growing extremely anxious, witnessing drastic changes in her once-kind, quiet, conscientious husband.

Along with acting uninterested in work, Harold was waking up screaming with nightmares. He was sometimes talking in a meaningless jumble. He was suspicious my mother was being unfaithful, and that both she and some restaurants may be poisoning his food.

As my body lay in its crib, my mother says my dad sometimes made ritualistic arm gestures over it, almost like the sign of the Christian cross (he was not a churchgoer). It made my mom worry he was going to slice me up. He would also scare my mother by holding her throat and talking about how pretty it was.

Eventually, he waved a knife at her. That was the turning point. My mom felt she had no choice. Calling the police was the only way, in those days, that an unwilling person with psychiatric illness could get treatment. It often still is today.

When the police arrived to take my father away, my mom felt incredibly guilty. In her anxiety, she wondered if maybe she *had* been a bad wife. She could hardly bear her sadness as she watched her once mild-mannered husband, at age twenty-eight, run down the street to escape the chasing police.

He stayed in Riverview for the next eighteen years. In the first few months he was angry and uncooperative and diagnosed as paranoid schizophrenic, though he didn't appear to be hearing voices (a key symptom of the disease).

He was soon subjected to scores of electroshock and lithium coma treatments (the latter were banned soon after). They seemed to accomplish nothing, other than to fry parts of his brain. I'm not necessarily blaming anyone, since ignorance and confusion abounded about psychoses. I'm sure most hospital staff sincerely wanted to help. Still, over the next many years, while Riverview psychiatrists tried different medications to stabilize my dad, Harold learned to simply do what he was told: be passive. It's known as being "institutionalized."

Meanwhile, back home, after the police caught my dad, my panicked mom called her brother, my Uncle George, to pick us up. We went to live with him and my grandmother in East Vancouver. Mom began working at Vulcan Automotive Equipment Ltd. as a secretary, remaining there the rest of her working life, bringing in the money to raise us. My devastated grandparents eventually realized their son was ill and did everything they could to help.

Despite the stigma, family and neighbours pitched in to support my mother and help raise my brother and me. Gratitude to them will always be eternal. Since people seemed to go out of their way to be friendly and not talk to me about my dad's illness, our lives appeared almost normal—if you didn't count the regular Sunday visits to Riverview Mental Hospital.

■   ■   ■

As an adult, I continued the tradition of Sunday visits with my father, although I certainly didn't do so every week as I did when I was a child.

I'd take Harold to parks for walks, to baseball games, to restaurants, and to the horse races, anything that would provide distraction. I occasionally asked my sons to come along because their grandfather is a part of the family history. Call it loyalty.

I learned to have no expectations on these excursions. So, when my dad did say something, it would be a bonus. Occasionally, he'd talk about the Vancouver Canucks hockey team or something in the news. A bit of a square, his favourite TV show was *Lawrence Welk*, the same as his parents.

During our visits he'd occasionally smile or chuckle to himself, appreciating some inner joke that was a complete mystery to me.

I knew some people would discreetly stare at him. But, for the most part, I tried not to care.

After many years at Riverview, Harold had been able to move out and live for a while with his parents, where we went to see him for Sunday dinners. As my grandparents became frail and eventually died, Harold ended up in a provincial government–run boarding house in the Vancouver neighbourhood of Kitsilano, not far from where he grew up.

Since I lived in the same area, I'd see him occasionally as he regularly walked the neighbourhood or visited libraries. He'd wear good leather shoes (his only luxury) and often a businessman's-style raincoat.

It was a bit of a shock to see him in public, say from across a street, the way a stranger would. I'd have to remind myself, "That man is my father." Like many offspring of mentally ill parents, I sometimes wondered if I was actually someone else's son. To me, he looked totally foreign: an alone and withdrawn figure from some sort of primeval world. For some reason his masklike face reminded me of a hawk.

Yet, although Harold looked "different" and rarely spoke, he was orderly, never smoked, read the *Vancouver Sun* newspaper, and the rotating staff at his boarding house generally saw him as a quiet man who was easy to get along with. Some called him a "gentleman." As he aged, his antipsychotic medications had been reduced to minute doses.

Over the years, several mental-health specialists who knew about my father had suggested he may have been misdiagnosed as schizophrenic, since it was a blanket label used for almost anyone with mental problems in the 1950s.

They speculated my dad's breakdown might have been caused by post-traumatic stress disorder, related to witnessing the brutalities of the Second World War at the tender age of eighteen. I was drawn to the theory, in part because it would have lifted some of the worries for me about my three sons. I not only didn't want to see them stigmatized by the disease, I would have preferred not to worry they had slightly greater odds than members of the general population about being genetically predisposed to it.

To get to the bottom of the horrible puzzle, I obtained my father's medical records from Riverview Hospital. While the records suggest most of his years of treatment were benignly ineffective, he was also "punished" in the first years by being sent as a "guest" to a closed ward. His crime: "a lack of interest and reluctance to work" in the hospital laundry.

Two friends, who were psychiatrists, once reviewed the records and cautiously concluded, even though it wasn't necessarily what I wanted to hear, that Harold, indeed, probably had suffered schizophrenic episodes. In response, I told myself that almost all children have at least one ancestor who suffered from a genetically linked disease. I also reminded myself that life is risky. (And, anyway, my growing kids seem more than fine.)

Reading my dad's medical records, it hit home that the main difference between then and now is, if my dad had exhibited the same symptoms today as he did in the 1950s, modern advances in medicine and medication would have made his chances of recovery and living a decent life much, much higher.

I've had to grieve that my dad was among the severely unlucky ones, in part because he was simply born at the wrong time. I'm not proud of it, but I felt his life was a waste. And the repercussions of his illness and treatment had spread well beyond him. My mother basically never talked about his breakdown, saying later she couldn't bear the pain of remembering. Some might suggest she acted unusually cheerful, as an understandable defence. My brother and I were, I think, scarred with deep-rooted shame and wariness about human existence and its many dangers. On the positive side, perhaps, all of us in the family developed a heightened sense of compassion for those who suffer.

That said, something happened in the mid-1990s that was remarkable, at least to me.

I was having lunch with work colleagues at Picasso's Restaurant on Broadway in Vancouver when I saw some artwork on the walls. Some of the paintings were signed, "Harold Todd." Stunned, I said, "That's my father's name."

The Kitsilano Mental Health team staff, it turned out, had convinced my dad to take an art workshop. Almost every week for a year or two he'd been painting his childlike patterns. Diffident to the extreme, he hadn't told us.

The Kitsilano Mental Health team staff had even helped him sell some. My brother and I now display some of his art in our houses. One painting in my study depicts a patchwork of red look-alike homes (perhaps like the one my dad was never really able to live in).

In a fragile way, my dad was blossoming, expressing himself.

Later, on another Sunday outing, when Harold was seventy-four, he again quietly shocked me.

He actually suggested where he'd like to go for lunch. Resigned to his utter passivity, this was the first time in forty-five years that I remembered him expressing a distinct preference. He asked to go to The Cactus Club Cafe on Broadway near Granville. I have no idea why he chose this trendy, flashy place. I figured it couldn't be the restaurant's voluptuous female servers in tight black uniforms. But you never know.

A couple of months after lunch at the Cactus Club I got a call from the kindly Filipina woman who ran Harold's boarding house. My dad had suffered a major heart attack and was in the Vancouver General Hospital. I found out later he'd been having pains in his arms and chest but had thought they were minor and wouldn't visit his general practitioner. My dad had great capacity for suffering in silence.

The hospital's attending doctor didn't think it was worth coming to the ward to talk to me in person, however. Over the phone the physician (whom I am tempted to name, in retaliation) said she wouldn't make any special effort to treat Harold's heart problems because, after all, he was a schizophrenic. He had, she said, virtually no quality of life.

I admit a part of me could see the doctor's chilling logic. But another part of me was raging. I wanted to shake the doctor into some semblance of humanity—at least show her my dad was capable of creating alluring paintings. About an hour after this phone conversation, however, following a severe convulsion of pain, Harold died as I held his hand. It was October 14, 1999.

Good friends, family, and some people from Harold's art class and boarding house came to his funeral. We displayed some of his paintings, the leather shoes he liked so much to walk in, and a photo of his immaculate bedroom, which looked like it could have housed a monk.

My brother and I said a few words about our dad. In his simple, stoic way, he had had a life. But the stigma of schizophrenia had pressed down on him to the moment of his death.

Lessons from Uncle Charles

JENNIFER CROWDER

When it arrived ten years ago, I almost missed it—a handwritten letter addressed to me, hidden among the usual stack of unsolicited mail. I instantly recognized the sender, whose penmanship resembles my father's but has ascenders that veer up and right with a hint of melodrama. I could recite the contents of its first paragraph—his standard opening—by heart:

> How, are, you, getting, along, today? I, am, well, and, getting, along, fine, here, in, Denver. I, expect, to, have, a, good, day. I, *should*, have, a, good, day!
>
> I, am, pleased, you, are, coming, to, Denver, for, a, conference! I, would, like, you, to, visit, me, here, at, Exeter, House, on, June, 16, at, 7, PM. I, will, pray, for, your, safe, travel, to, Denver!

He concluded with his full name: "Sincerely, Charles V. Adams." I'm sure he has never considered another signature—one shorter and less formal for personal notes. Charles V. Adams is his legal name, so that's the signature he always uses.

Years ago, Uncle Charles used fewer commas. He has always prided himself on his command of grammar, especially punctuation. He likes punctuation—he's probably drawn to its precision and lack of ambiguity. His sentences end with bold, large periods that stand out in relief on the back of the paper like Braille and say, unequivocally, *Stop here!* His commas are similarly definitive, dark arcs that resemble a flock of birds poised to rise from the page.

But why after every word? I've tried many times to imagine my way into my uncle's mind, yet his thoughts and motivations remain elusive. I'm certain Charles was troubled when the rules of grammar began to become more fluid. Charles dislikes change, and the sudden ambiguity about the use of serial commas must have bothered him intensely. He probably felt betrayed to the point of adopting his own comma policy: the more, the better. Since then, he has surely noticed that letters arriving from others have fewer commas than his own. But he remains steadfast. He, at least, is consistent.

Uncle Charles is my father's only sibling and four years his senior. He has lived for more than thirty years in a Denver "assisted living guest home," supported by the Veterans Administration. He has been diagnosed as schizophrenic.

Uncle Charles first enlisted in the air force in 1953 and successfully served one tour of duty in Korea. He re-enlisted in 1958 but left the air force less than a year later following a major psychological breakdown in Greenland, where he'd been stationed at Thule Air Force Base. Although the military flew him back to the States, to New Jersey, for some reason—a terrible error? Negligence? Mere indifference?—he was released there rather than being taken on to his home in Colorado.

Charles disappeared and didn't resurface until four weeks later, when he called his parents from a New York City payphone. My grandfather flew there to pick him up. All we know about that month is that it seems to mark decisively the beginning of his fully developed mental illness. I'm not sure anyone has ever asked him what happened. I can't bring myself to do it; I worry about the potential consequences of even referring to this part of his life. The most I can do is to speculate—to construct a fictional account of those lost days in New York and the interval in Greenland that preceded them.

■ ■ ■

The August Manhattan streets simmer beneath his feet as he is carried through the tide of people—all strangers, so many!—like a boat that has slipped its mooring and floated into unfamiliar waters. Noise assaults him—a dissonant mix of car horns, shrieking tires, people shouting, and the constant drumming of footsteps on pavement.

In Greenland, Charles spent days on end in the Communications Center monitoring the Teletype. Though he occasionally saw others, he felt entombed in the intense silence. But the howling Arctic gales were worse. They awoke him at night, racing over the expanses of ice and rock, whipping up clouds of snow and sliding beneath his door with an insidious hiss that whispered to him like judgment.

■ ■ ■

Ten years ago, I was working on a corporate web team in Seattle and learned that I would be attending a conference in Denver. I remember thinking, *I should visit Uncle Charles.* But I hesitated. Spending time with him is not easy. His disease, combined with his medications, frequently make him remote. To have a conversation with him, you must initiate and sustain it. He rarely makes eye contact. When he speaks, it's likely to be on a topic unrelated to anything you've been saying.

Still, I told myself, *he's alone there, and my uncle.* Our family is small, and he has just two nieces and two nephews, all then living on the West Coast. He rarely has visitors. More than mere obligation, I felt a certain affection for him. I've always trusted his good intentions and knew he was doing his best.

My feelings toward him weren't always so charitable. As children, my sister, twin brothers, and I didn't understand our uncle. Though my parents tried to explain that he was different from most other adults and emphasize understanding and tolerance, we couldn't appreciate the nature of his illness.

When we were young, we found considerable humour in Uncle Charles. The classic incident occurred the summer our grandfather—who taught us to fish and tied beautiful fishing flies with captivating names such as the Copper John and the Mickey Finn—took us trout fishing on the banks of the Arkansas River just upstream from the Royal Gorge. Uncle Charles, then living at home, decided to join us. We received that news without enthusiasm. We thought he was weird.

Uncle Charles has the most prominent version of the Adams nose. In retrospect, it seems inevitable that he would become the target of a wayward fly that sought refuge in one of his nostrils. He reacted predictably, with a spectacular display of snorting, gasping, and frantic attempts to extricate the intruder. We found it hilarious—far more exciting even than a fireworks show—and laughed ourselves silly. Embarrassed and angry, he fumed all afternoon.

Later, when maturity granted us a measure of sensitivity, we usually managed to avoid laughing at Uncle Charles directly. Instead, we snickered among ourselves about his oddities. Chief among these was his taste in clothing. His signature outfit combined a suit coat, pants, vest, and tie, all with clashing plaids in varying shades of maroon. Fortunately, whenever he appeared in dubious ensembles, my mother intervened and diplomatically helped him choose other attire.

■　■　■

Charles sits at his station, watching a mind-numbing stream of words and characters spill from the Teletype. Suddenly he frowns and leans in for a closer look. The words seem to shimmer on the printout, like the surface of a lake disturbed by a gust of wind. Is he imagining it? He peers at the tape. Soon, characters and whole words begin sliding to the edges of the spooled paper, then falling onto the cement floor in an indecipherable tangle.

Perspiration shines on his brow and a rivulet of cold sweat traces an irregular path down his cheek. His breathing quickens and becomes ragged. What was that last message? Perhaps the radars on the new DEW Line have detected a Soviet attack! Charles drops to the floor, the Teletype paper coiling around him like a snake. He snatches up the word *launching*, then looks left and right for *missile*, his hands shaking violently as he sifts through the jumbled words.

■   ■   ■

Charles likely has never considered whether or not he is a good uncle. But he writes to his nieces and nephews faithfully, rarely forgetting to send birthday and seasonal cards, often a month early. He visits us in Seattle annually, usually during the holidays. My father makes flight reservations, and Charles relies on his comprehensive knowledge of the Denver bus system to get to the airport on the appointed day and time. He arrives hours early, his single suitcase meticulously packed and his watch preset to Pacific Standard Time by appointment the previous day with a neighbourhood jeweller. He is devoted to us in his own detached, earnest way.

When I finally arrive in Denver for the conference and the day of my visit with Uncle Charles is at hand, he occupies my thoughts all morning. As I sit through forgettable presentations, I envision Charles's standard morning routine, which proceeds at a glacial pace. He's extraordinarily deliberate, often struggling to decide what to wear. When he finally makes a choice, he lays out the selected articles of clothing on the bed in a specific manner and sequence. If this ritual is disrupted, his anxiety spikes quickly— he cannot even look at his clothes, much less distinguish a shirt from a pair of socks. He sits on the edge of the bed, frowning and muttering to himself until one of my parents arrives to intervene.

It occurs to me that my own visit will be a huge disruption to Charles's routine, and I wonder uneasily how it might affect him. But I've already committed to going, and he's expecting me.

I'll need to carry any conversation we have, so I mull over what we might talk about. Uncle Charles has decided opinions about politics, and the absolute views of the conservative right are immensely appealing to him. In recent letters, he has expressed grave concern about "foreigners." He worries that they're "taking over the country, depriving hard working Americans of good jobs." He hears inflammatory speeches about the "immigrant invasion" at a monthly Denver Chapter meeting of the Republican National Committee. He proudly wears an RNC pin on his suit coat, along with pins that say, "AARP" and "*Jesus Saves!*" Each morning, he transfers the pins to the jacket he's chosen for the day.

Shortly after 9/11, the Denver RNC held a special event at Exeter House to honour the veterans living there. Uncle Charles sent us a copy of the program, which listed his name and service dates as a Korean War veteran. In his accompanying letter, he proclaimed himself "Proud, to, be, an, American!" coincidentally the event's theme. Thereafter, he concluded all conversations—whether with family, friends, or waitresses—with the heartfelt declaration, "God Bless America!"

▪ ▪ ▪

Charles has been ordered to return to the States. The papers refer to a "Medical Discharge"—why? He vaguely recalls being in the Teletype room, the hum of the machines, and characters and words in disarray on the floor. A sense of falling, then a fracture, followed by—nothing. Whatever happened leaves his mind blank, empty. He's aware of having lost time. He can't order his thoughts; he tries to write a letter to his parents but can't make the pen move on the paper.

He sits in a C-130 near a pallet of supply boxes, ears ringing from the roar of the propellers. Distant voices and an occasional burst of laughter echo from somewhere ahead of him, but he can't see anyone or distinguish individual words. He strains to see beyond the tepid beam of daylight that has insinuated itself through the tiny, streaked window. He can just make out the sea far below. He tries to pray but gets no further than, "God, where's Colorado Springs?"

■　■　■

Later that afternoon, as I set off through rush hour traffic for downtown Denver, I wonder if my parents should bring Uncle Charles to Seattle. I know they've agonized over that question. He can't live independently; he'd probably burn up an apartment. He can forget for days to shower or launder his clothes. His naivety about money makes him extremely vulnerable—an unscrupulous salesman who learned of his interest in photography once nearly succeeded in selling him an industrial camera costing nearly ten thousand dollars. Fortunately, my father caught on in time and stopped the sale. Since then, he's managed my uncle's finances.

Uncle Charles's ubiquitous presence during the holidays can be oppressive—just being with him, sustaining a conversation, takes considerable effort and emotional energy, especially when he's overmedicated and remote. Yet when Uncle Charles is at his best—at odd, unexpected moments—he can be delightful. One Christmas, my brothers received the game Trivial Pursuit as a gift. Just as the four of us sat down to play for the first time, Uncle Charles appeared in the doorway. Reluctantly, we invited him to join us. We assumed he'd bog down the action. To our surprise, he handily smoked us all, displaying an astounding memory for facts of all sorts. That night, he was engaged, an active participant with a funny *haw haw* laugh and a genuine smile. We later agreed the best part of the evening was hearing his laugh—we weren't sure we ever had before. At these rare moments, we catch fleeting glimpses of the person he might have been if not ill, if his personality hadn't been smothered by pharmaceuticals.

We all work hard to evoke these moments, teasing him and making jokes. It is so immensely satisfying, so surprising, when we succeed in temporarily drawing him out. Usually, though, we don't. And our successes are becoming rarer as Uncle Charles ages.

■ ■ ■

Charles stops in the plane's doorway, blinking in the bright sunlight. *Where am I?* he wonders just as he's shoved from behind by an impatient airman. He spots a sign: Welcome to McGuire Air Force Base! He tries to comprehend why he's here, but his mind feels detached, shrouded.

In an airless office, he accepts papers thrust into his hands by an officious staff sergeant. He pockets the papers without reading them and follows others through a door, which opens onto a busy corridor. Military personnel stream by. He's immediately caught up like flotsam and swept outside to an area where several buses wait curbside. He feels a surge of hope: "Mother and Dad will be here!" He searches the crowd for a familiar face but sees none.

■ ■ ■

Shortly before 7:00 PM, I arrive at Exeter House. I study the mid-sized, two-storey white building that occupies most of a city block. The bare branches of the trees around its periphery etch a lacy pattern in the evening sky. A broad porch with a sparse assortment of mismatched lawn chairs spans the front. It's a bit derelict but seems welcoming enough, with half its windows lit. The building looks to be about 1920s vintage and probably began life as a hotel or apartment building.

I'm uneasy about what I'll find inside. I've never visited a home like this. Are all the residents mentally ill? Are they medicated and under control like my uncle? If they're not, are they restrained? *But my father's been here*, I assure myself. If he had any concerns about my safety while visiting, I know he'd have shared them.

As I lock the car door, I hear a loud "Hello, Jennifer!" and see Uncle Charles waving from the front porch. As we exchange the usual awkward hug, I'm surprised to see tears in his eyes. I'm suddenly *very* glad I came. What I've been regarding as a casual visit means a tremendous amount to him. I'm chagrined that I've been so cavalier about the evening, treating it so lightly. From Charles's perspective, I'm the first of his brother's children to visit him here in thirty years. *Thirty years.*

Most of Uncle Charles's abundant, once-dark hair is now steely grey. He's peering out of the same horrible glasses he's worn for years, and I resolve to persuade my father to help him find an updated pair during his next visit.

"Ahhh . . ." he begins and runs his tongue over his lips as he opens and closes his mouth repeatedly, fishlike, a familiar nervous habit. He looks at me expectantly, like an actor unsure whether he's heard his cue yet.

"Uncle Charles! It's so good to see you! And finally to see your home!"

"Yes! It's fine to see you too. I prayed today for your safe travel, and . . ." He breaks off, uncertain what to say next.

I take his arm, smiling.

"I'm glad you did. Thanks to you, I had a safe trip. I'm hoping for a tour of the home before we go out. I'd love to see your room so I can picture you here when I'm back in Seattle. And I bet you have some great new photos."

"*Yes*, yes, I have," Charles nods vigorously, his tone definitive. "I will show you the home and introduce you to my friends. And we will look at my latest photos!"

In the lobby, I meet Glynis, the evening front desk attendant. Her luminous blond hair is startling on a woman I guess to be in her seventies. But she seems warm and kind.

As Charles and I walk through the hallways, I'm aware of being studied closely by the residents we pass and the few to whom I'm introduced. Yet I never feel threatened. Instead, I have a sense of delayed action, as if Exeter House operates in a parallel universe where time passes more slowly and is measured differently, in increments unfamiliar to the rest of the world.

On the second floor, we stop outside a nondescript door, no different from any of the others we've passed. "This is my room," Charles announces as he turns a key in the lock.

I'm not sure what I'd expected, but my overwhelming impression is of a lifetime distilled into one small space. Like a time capsule. The furnishings are spare: I see a neatly made bed and matching dresser, a small writing desk and chair by the room's single window, an armchair, and an aged TV. But the room overflows with tokens of family—the afghan my sister crocheted for his sixtieth birthday, pictures I coloured in grade school, bookends we'd sent one Christmas. On the dresser top sits a dish with a scratched and faded image of Old Faithful, above a banner exclaiming "Magnificent Yellowstone!" I remember sending it to him after a family vacation years ago.

But mainly photos, everywhere, almost entirely of our family. Fading school photos of my sister and me, more than thirty years old. Photos from family trips. Holiday photos. Even a few framed prints of Charles and my father with their parents when they were all much younger. His family, I realize, is his world.

I struggle to keep my voice even.

"It's a wonderful room, Uncle Charles. Very comfortable and warm."

"Yes," he replies, beaming.

As usual, Charles is eager to show off his latest photo album. As we leaf through the pages, I have a distinct sense of déjà vu, and realize that I've seen nearly all these photos before—kind of. The photographs show the same scenes but in different years. The same flowerbeds. The same trees in City Park, blanketed with spring flowers or blazing with autumn colour. Nearly identical views of the Denver zoo, the Museum of Nature and Science, the Civic Centre. In commas and photos alike, my uncle is nothing if not consistent. The photos are unremarkable, but he's clearly happy so I am patient. We look at every photo in the album.

We drive a short distance to a restaurant Uncle Charles likes and order pie and coffee. We talk a little more, though he's tired and begins to retreat into himself. Soon the limited conversation we've managed to sustain up to now ends. I drive him back to Exeter House and see him into the lobby, where I give him another hug, thank him for the evening, and bid him goodnight.

"God Bless America!" he calls as the door closes.

Back in the car, I sit with my hands on the steering wheel and watch steam form on the cold windshield. The visit went better than I'd expected and I'm relieved. Although Uncle Charles is one of the home's oldest residents and doesn't have a lot of friends, the few I've met that evening seem like good people. He's not alone there. Still, I'm again near tears as I realize it may be years before I'm in Denver again. It saddens me to imagine my uncle here without family nearby, leading his modest, quiet life. But there's no ideal alternative. He knows this city; it's home. And, I remind myself, he's fortunate to have a safe and reliable residence. Many vets are on the streets. He is a good, kind man. He is conscientious and honourable. *I am fortunate to be his niece*, I think to myself. And I'm surprised that I've just realized that.

■ ■ ■

Charles stands alone in Times Square, overwhelmed by the dizzying motion of the supersized billboards that tower over him. He dimly remembers the bus from McGuire and the brusque cabbie who drove him here, the only place Charles could name in this city. Images flash with neon insistence and letters race across one of the billboards, too fast for him to catch. More Teletype messages? What warning might they contain? He shivers as the daylight begins to fade and the wind picks up. It's a summer breeze, but Charles cannot feel its warmth, pursued still by the Arctic chill of his nightmares. He backs up against the wall of a building and sinks to the ground, his hands grasping each side of his head. People rush past, their gazes fixed resolutely elsewhere.

■ ■ ■

I return to Denver sooner than I'd expected, accompanying my mother to her mother's memorial service. My maternal grandmother, Mildred, was nearly ninety-nine when she passed away.

The morning of the service, we awake to find more than a foot of new snow on the ground. It is beautiful, but I know it will keep many older family members and friends at home, afraid to drive. So we expect the small service to be sparsely attended.

We leave early to prepare for the 9:30 AM service. Reaching the cemetery gates at barely 8:00 AM, we're surprised to find we aren't the first to arrive. A single set of footprints precedes us on the road curving through the gravestones to the chapel where the memorial is to be held.

Opening the chapel door, we find Uncle Charles sitting calmly on a bench in the hallway, dressed warmly and wearing galoshes. He stands, smiling, and greets us.

"But how did you get here?" my mother asks. We know Exeter House is on the other side of the city.

"I took the bus," states Uncle Charles. His matter-of-fact tone makes clear that he sees nothing extraordinary about his presence here. We later learn he has taken three buses, the first of them just after 5:30 AM, to get here. We're stunned. He has made this trip to honour his sister-in-law's mother.

It probably never occurred to him to do otherwise. To Uncle Charles, my mother's mother is part of his family. And family, more than anything else, defines the boundaries of his world and informs his values and choices. In a world he often finds confusing and overwhelming, family is the language he understands best—one uninterrupted by commas and impervious to distance. Family is his safe harbour, his touchstone, his source of meaning and satisfaction. And for that I have tremendous respect.

Hindsight

ERIN HART MacNAIR

I put the phone down with a gentle click. My eyes feel ruined, gouged. I push both palms into them, hoping the pressure will soothe the ache. I force my wrists upward to erase pain with more pain. Red and yellow sunspots flash in the darkness. We had shared the same blue eyes, shared the same intense, steely-grey flash when we were angry. When we were angry, past tense. Had he done this? Had he wiped tears away from his sea-blue stunners or were they ice-cold flint, set in grim determination? In a flash of noise and violence, it suddenly didn't matter. He destroyed the windows to his soul at the beck and call of a manic man's God. I am thirty-one, and my father has just killed himself.

■ ■ ■

I am seven, and the things that matter most to me now are family, friends, and my new sneakers.

"Go ahead, touch it," Dad said, smiling down at me. I stared at the lifeless body of a rainbow trout, shimmering under the fluorescent lights of our basement workshop. I ease out my index finger as his fillet knife makes a grating, swishing sound as he sharpens it.

Dad pulls at one of my red braids. "Go on." I poked at the eyeball, oily and viscous beneath my finger. I ran my finger over the lifeless orb, ripe in its fishy stink, griming up the newspaper it lay upon. I jabbed a bit farther, digging into the cavity behind the eye, lifting it slightly. Dad motioned for me to move, and I scooted to the tail end of the fish. "Here is how it's done." He sliced into the delicate flesh, folding back a layer of scales and grease. Eggs slipped out of the bottom half and I made a face.

"But it's a mom!" I cried.

He cautiously looked my way. "We try to not catch the moms, but sometimes it happens." I stared at the eggs, silent. Dad scraped them into a plastic-lined bin and continued carving bits of unwanted flesh from the supple meat. Why was it better to catch the dads? I wondered. Are dads somehow less important? Mine wasn't, not to me. I held him in childlike awe for most of my youth: he was funnier, smarter, and larger than everyone else's dad. He was handsome and tall, with wiry dark hair and large, bearlike hands. A salesman, he was gone four or five days of the week, which only increased my idolization of him. He must be really important, I thought, to be away so much of the time. And he had super-human powers, like staying up for days on end without any sleep. He had an infectious, booming laugh and a nervous tic that made him silently repeat words he had said. Especially the funny words, *funny words, funny words*.

Each day with Dad was different. Some days he was a jovial, brilliant man, other times he was quiet, aloof, and grouchy. Manic depression breeds fast learners in children, and my brother and I would signal to each other if the day was a "bear day" or a regular dad day. I would sneak downstairs and poke my head around the corner, checking his lair. His posture, his knit eyebrows, and his fidgeting all told me how the day was going to go. I learned to read the signs, and the signs often said "Keep away." I didn't have any real understanding of the impact on my mom. She was nervous and tense, I knew that much. They were married at eighteen, and her new husband was mentally ill at twenty. My mom was basically a single mother.

Manic depression didn't mar our childhood: it skirted the edges of our lives like a burnt rim on a beautiful cake. We had no idea what a "normal" family was like, so ours was by all means normal. Our dad was fun; he was silly and did ridiculous things. Once he turned off the highway into a cornfield to make a U-turn. My brother and I squealed with delight from the back seat of our hand-painted, bright blue station wagon. "Yyyeeeeehaawwww!" he whooped, popping back onto the highway with only a scattering of corn ears to say where we'd been. The exhilaration of blatant rule-breaking was infectious; that was just one of many moments that made us love him.

Then, he would go missing. Mom would say he'd be away for a while, on a "long work trip." She couldn't say when he'd be back. We never thought to question, never paused to see the patterns that snaked though our lives seasonally.

Finally she had to tell us.

She nervously shifted on the couch in the living room, picking at the edge of a pillow. The story emerged in bits and pieces, the latest piece first. I was a wilful thirteen, my brother sixteen. "That time last winter, well, he was in the hospital, taking the lithium he was supposed to take daily." This new incident was serious, he had been to jail. He had beaten up some policemen when they prevented him from trying to "talk" to a country music star. It took eight policemen to take him down. They zapped him with stun guns countless times before he succumbed. Later she would tell me how she screamed at them, "He's ill! He needs medication, he's not well, for chrissake!" I pictured her screaming, her frail hands grabbing at them, her face contorted with fear. My mother has aged prematurely.

Paul and I sat in heavy silence. How could we not have seen this? How could they not have told us? I felt betrayed, lied to. I stroked the fraying ends of the carpeting on which I sat, trying to hide my anger. It didn't take long for the questions to boil out of us. Then Mom was upright, pillow tossed aside. She was ready for us. This woman had been through a lot of shit and now we were going to give her some more, with a mixture of teenaged venom and incomprehension thrown in. The puzzle pieces clicked into place. I got it now. This illness explained the angry and silent man, the happy and enthusiastic one. When there was nothing left to clarify, I stumbled to my room. I cranked on the radio and lay back on my bed. I stared up at the ceiling and waited for the world to cave in.

The house became divided with invisible walls. Paul and I sensed the imminent divorce and made plans to move out and move on. Immediately after my brother graduated from high school, Dad moved to a different town, a girlfriend waiting in the wings. Paul followed him there, a bit lost and directionless. He moved close to Dad to be near him, but also to watch over him, hiding the truth from me. He once stayed up with Dad for almost forty hours, talking him down off a high Dad had placed a handgun on the coffee table and would periodically pick it up to emphasize a point. He raved about God and angels, how we were chosen people, how we would survive the imminent Armageddon. Paul eventually got him to the hospital. Afterwards Paul was ever watchful, keeping one eye on the door at family gatherings. Hearing this really pissed me off. Why did my young brother feel he had to defend the fort? Where were all the adults?

Paul and I had numerous late-night pep talks, trying to hash out the details of Dad's illness, weighing the odds of suicide. We readied ourselves by asking, "What'll you do if, when . . ."

As I got older, my dad and I held a steady course of one step forward, three steps backwards. We'd engage in long conversations about how we felt the world worked, from physics to spirituality. We pontificated on inner intimacies and felt like observers of unseen forces. We had a psychic connection that was uncanny. I didn't have manic depression, but I had extreme bouts of melancholy that had at least once bordered on suicide. He said he knew how I felt, and that we shared a "gift," the gift of deep feeling and connection to this Earth. He explained that this gift was a blessing and a burden, as it would pain us like the weight Atlas bore. Our understanding of each other was incredibly intense, which made our falling-outs painful to bear. He'd call at five in the morning to trounce me with something I'd said when I was fifteen, some slight I'd offered him or his new wife. One minute we were holding steady, the next, I was on top of the shit list. These ups and downs threw me. I knew what the illness was about, knew its painful narcissistic tendencies. Yet I couldn't bring myself to steel my emotions, as my brother had. As I aged, I discovered ways. Distance was one of them, and I found myself halfway around the world when the call came.

You can't prepare yourself for that call. The shock of it made me sick, and I ran to the bathroom, throwing the phone at my husband. He talked to my mom as I tried to quiet myself, absorb the wave of emotions. In the still moments afterwards, my body purged, I felt relief. He had escaped his illness. I pictured my dad, throwing me in the air and laughing, my braids hanging in weightless space as I shrieked with happiness.

I splashed cold water on my face and stared into the mirror. The call had finally come, but I wouldn't have to dread it any longer. Wherever Dad was, he would have to look through my eyes now.

Flying Wounded

SUSAN McCASLIN

Mom raises two children in the suburbs of Indianapolis in the 1950s and Seattle in the 1960s. In 1963, she has a "nervous breakdown." Throughout her life, she experiences dramatic mood swings that, nowadays, would lead to a diagnosis of bipolar disorder. In the early 1960s, her doctor prescribes diet pills laced with amphetamines. Later, I come across an article published in the early 1970s that indicates this particular drug has been taken off the market for inducing schizophrenia in women all across America.

After taking the diet pills, Mom begins experiencing hallucinations and delusions of a religious nature. When I am sixteen, she descends into a catatonic state and is conveyed forcibly to a nearby university hospital. There she is treated with experimental, hallucinogenic drugs that the doctors later admit pushed her further into psychosis. After several months of treatment, she is released and advised to remain on medication for the rest of her life. Immediately she flushes the meds down the toilet and refuses to ever see a doctor again. Mom never recovers from her midlife trauma.

■　■　■

Leaky Condoms and Early Discomfort Zones

My grandfather's hardware store in Albertville, Alabama, goes bankrupt during the Depression when my mother is twelve. Soon Mom and her family move up north to Indianapolis, where she attends high school.

When she and her brother near university age, her folks move north to Lafayette, where they can afford to send the kids to Purdue University. Purdue is mainly an engineering college at the time where one of the only disciplines open to women is "Home Economics." Though Mom doesn't see herself as the domestic type, she finds herself turning out perfect lemon meringue pies in a state-of-the-art campus kitchen. Soon she meets my dad, a handsome boarder in her parents' home, but shows little interest in him. My grandmother keeps pushing her to invite this six-foot five-inch, shy, lanky lad to the Sadie Hawkins because he seems "so sweet" and because he props a photograph of his parents on his desk. "Any boy who honours his parents like that just has to be a fine young man," my grandmother quips. A few dates later, Mom agrees to become engaged. Soon the bombs fall on Pearl Harbor, Dad signs up for the air force, my parents marry, and he heads off to the Philippines. When the war ends, they settle into a suburb of Indianapolis.

Mom isn't sure she is prepared to have children so puts off the issue indefinitely. Dad, whose whole notion of marriage is that children will ensue quickly, grumbles while she stalls. Years later, she discloses she once caught him sitting on the bed determinedly poking pinholes in a condom. It is shortly afterwards in 1947 that she becomes pregnant and gives birth to me, followed, again reluctantly, by my brother in 1952.

Letting Herself Go

into harpy, medusa
midnight ice cream reveler

Mom balloons out
puffing and huffing

exchanges her smart clothes
and dyed-to-match shoes

for mismatched patchwork robes,
cuts her hair in jagged strips,

indulges screaming fits, occasionally
fixes herself in hall mirrors

(still lipsticked and smiling),
then begins to say the unsayable

to whoever wants or does not
want to hear.

"It has finally comes to this,"
she hears her mother say,

"She has let herself go."

Grooving into the 1960s

Mom is manic during my childhood—buying sprees, constant fights
with my dad, screaming matches, and flying fry pans. My small back
bedroom becomes a citadel of order against chaos where I turn to
fairy tales and excerpts from the classics in children's anthologies.
There I slip into alternative worlds of enchantment. My father,
realist, oddball, underdog, but more stable than Mom, has no idea
how to cope with her extreme mood swings. "Just straighten up
and fly right," he seems to be saying. Steady provider, housekeeper,
and cook, he becomes for me a stabilizing presence and I a "Dad's
girl." It takes me decades to realize how much of my anxiety over
loss of control stems from my response to my mother's emotional
instability; yet I also realize my idealization of my father reveals
only part of the story. I know now that Mom was out of place in this

standardized 1950s bastion of conformity, her own imagination and intelligence stifled.

Dad, dissatisfied with his job as an engineer at General Motors, is offered a job at Boeing in 1959, so we fly to Seattle, full of hope for new beginnings. The incessant fighting intensifies, even before we move from a motel to a nicer, larger home in a new subdivision. During my high school years, when I become preoccupied with grades and singled out as a promising young poet by one of my teachers, Mom's pre-menopausal years arrive along with her religious obsessions and delusions.

Devil's Eyes and Voices

One day she is reading the Bible
and all the pertinent texts
raise themselves in yellow light;
filaments of words grow fat with meaning
and a fleshy wing circumscribes her
like a wind. There is a whirring
and she rolls like Ezekiel on her side
acting God's rejection and love for Israel.

Her teenage daughter enters the room
wearing emerald eye shadow slanting up
at the corners. Green eyes smirk.

It's the devil wearing green,
old fool, and her daughter has been
whisked away on a wing and a prayer.

The voices begin chanting ditties,
issuing commands; the television
becomes vatic; ubiquitous eyes
murmur threats and promises.

She is finally at the centre of a world.

Proverbial White Coats

The crisis of my teens: Mom dragged away by men in white coats. A straitjacket with straps locks her arms tightly to her torso. That "coo-coo-a choo" chorus Simon and Garfunkel popularized about "Mrs. Robinson" comes out later, and I recognize the emotional landscape. Mom's absence those months leaves an unspeakable gap, frisson, the light from the window by her bed left in shards where her head had rested, restless on the pillow so many nights. When in university I tell my buddies, "My mom's just a little neurotic," I half believe that lie. One boyfriend, after meeting her, sneers, "Your mom's a bubble head," and I take umbrage, breaking up with him right away—angry, protective. Years later, on showing my high school girlfriends some poems I had written about my mom's mental illness, they shake their heads, "None of us ever knew."

University Hospital

Thrown in a close cubical three days
you defecate on the floor
and no one comes to clean up;
only bland robotic leers
pierce through opaque cubes.

Sweet southern rose,
how your petals pour sweat
when they say you will never
see your children again
without co-operation
which means peeling
more therapeutic potatoes
and submitting to shots
(the drug of the month)
that send you somersaulting
further out into moonscapes
where we cannot, cannot come.

For three months
you tread that broken ward
where human detritus
shuffles and rocks
under priestly medicos
in their clean offices
on the seventh floor
who sometimes remove
their gloves when consulting.

Hammering Angels

Months after returning from the University Hospital, Mom tries to tell me what it was like. When she sprawled on the floor of a padded cell, her father came to visit several times but could only peer at her through a tiny portal. At first she thought his was the blue eye of God, then knew he was her father whom she adored, but they wouldn't let her see him. When the nurses brought her dinner on a tray, the voices said she could drink from the cup with the white straw but not the black, the latter being from the devil. The medicines made her mouth dry and her feet jittery.

One night she fell down on the floor of the cell and began to die. Everything darkened and she lost consciousness but awoke at the foot of a ladder and began to climb into the light. Partway up, someone asked if she wanted to go on to heaven or go back and be with her family. Instinctively, everything in her said *yes* to her earthly home. Immediately, a thousand hammers began rapping and tapping, firing silver sparks in her head that shimmered around the room. The pounding seemed to last forever but it felt quite pleasant. "What's happening?" she asked. The voice said the angels were fixing her head so she could go back to her children. A few days later word came that she would be going home.

On hearing these and other stories, part of me wants to experience what she endured. Part of me stands aside, numb and appalled. She is sick; she is untouchable; she is shamanic. Years later my writing becomes a way to retread these depths and heights. Looking back now, I wonder if my later investigations into the lives and writings of the mystics didn't originate here in our mutual need for self-transcendence.

Head Rifts

beyond the pale pale lady

"a great gulf fixed twixt
me and thee"

not a Lazarus tongue drop to unparch

we are us Laz are us
is us

Laser eye

yet I write wanting a centre
from which to scribe your lost body

while you explode quicksilver
my crazy Logos hold

words followed by
words words words
mouthed silently
Gestapo commands

It's one thing
to romanticize this craziness,
another to lurch
three months in hell
without a hand basket
(*worse than a Nazi
concentration camp*,
you said).

Just because you are paranoid, mother,
doesn't mean they aren't out to get you.

You heard at the gates of heaven
the angels' rat-a-tat hammers
repairing your brain.

If you could have gone higher
would you have heard them singing?

Crouching Teen, Sleeping Tiger

After she returns from the hospital and on through my late teens,
I spend my time avoiding her extremes. Mom's incessant in-your-
face chatter wears me out. Her constant offerings of Oreos and
coconut dream cake from Frederick & Nelson's bakery makes me
fatigued, as our blood sugars spike and plummet. She never seems
to grasp my love of books and academics, yet discourages sports and
boyfriends too. "Who can you trust?" "Why go skiing? You could
break a leg!"

She takes to gardening, napping, hiding behind fences, drinking
too many Manhattans and Brandy Alexanders at parties, then avoiding all social contact for months. Blinds close. She begins tacking
Bible quotes to walls and doors. I come home to a darkened house.
She plants bushes that, unpruned, gradually cover all the windows.

Teen in the Back Seat

Never say anything.
Scrunch back and let her
words rattle over you.

One wrong sound, one look
and honeyed titter whips itself
into hurricane; tornado mind
stops at nothing.

Just when she is most
hilarious, every sentence
punctuated by infectious chuckles,
most playful in her t-shirt

with the Garfield tea-towel
hand sewn on her chest,
and that chest rising
with side-splitting mirth

that is the moment
she dips down
(euphoric roller coaster plummeting)
where you (absolutely)
do not want to go.

Better let her winds
fluster themselves
and curl at last
to stupor.

Pigs, Snails, and Caterpillars

My mother has a fondness for animals and small creatures. When we
move from Indianapolis to Seattle, she packs Mittens, our black and
white cat, into a birdcage and grumbles at the men who shove him
roughly into the baggage compartment. Charlie, the cocker spaniel
rescued from the pound, immediately becomes "Mom's dog," but
after he dies of stomach cancer, she grieves for years, swearing she
will never ever again have a pet. Charlie's boon companion, Sammy
the cat, is fed tuna fish straight from the can until the day he dies.
After the "no more pet" rule is established, it is as if a signal goes
out over the neighbourhood—"All Derelicts and Strays Welcome!"

Years later when the man who is to become my husband meets
her, she leads him to the back porch, pointing to a collection of milk
cartons stacked beside the house. Inside each cut-open container is

a piece of lettuce or fruit. "Those are my snail apartments," she boasts. "The snails have everything they want, so they leave the flowers alone."

When Dad takes us in the car past a construction zone where large Caterpillar brand excavators squat row on row, she yells out: "'And your spoil shall be gathered like the gathering of the caterpillar': Isaiah 33:4!!!" Part of her is deadly serious about these apocalyptic signs, while another part chuckles at her own double entendre.

Ambivalent about her spirituality, I find that something in me wants to skip the craziness, the black and white thinking, the fears, yet absorb the sensitivity and compassion. Even today, Jain-like, in semblance of my mom, I will lift a ladybug or a gnat onto a napkin and place it gently in the garden rather than see it get washed down the drain or unceremoniously smashed.

Fatigued

Cushioned into your son's abandoned lower-bunk,
you hunker down for an all-day sleepathon.
Your light snoring fills the room
with hummingbird wings; you are sailing
away from morbid wakefulness.

Your body molds itself to sinuous cloud
and the cross on your brow unstiffens.
These days there is no incessant word-flow,
for almost always you are prostrate,
flattened, incomprehensible.

Jane Eyre and Bertha

After graduating from the University of Washington in English in 1969, I'm accepted into graduate school at Simon Fraser University in Canada. SFU, a hotbed of radicalism and radical poetics, attracts the left-wing, anti-Vietnam hippie-ish me, so my draft-resister boyfriend and I head across the border. Yet my avoidance-identification with my mother continues. I realize in retrospect that making my home in Canada is in part a way of placing an entire country between us. I experiment briefly with hallucinogenic drugs, partly out of a search for higher consciousness and partly out of a need to experience what she had known during her hallucinations. The novel *Jane Eyre* intrigues me because of Bertha, the madwoman in the attic Rochester hides from sweet, rational Jane. My mother is my own sort of madwoman in the attic whom I fear becoming—my dark secret other.

I Go Psychedelic for You (1969)

If poets are the antennae of the race
and allied with the compacted mad,
there is this compact, mother;
you shall go divinely insane
and I shall go behind you
wearing boa feathers and snakes

Jane Eyre and Bertha
(the madwoman in the attic)
reconciled; two big-time women
passing over the hill hilariously
into language, leagued
companions of the bipolar
disorder, delusions
and paranoias on poles
parading before.

Poets hear their voices too
and obey them just as religiously.

So I will go psychedelic for you mother
in floral skirts and chains
and wear green skippingly.

And when the interviewer asks,
"Is your mother still living?"
I shall answer, "Yes
I am."

Madness and Creativity

I think of my life as fairly conventional externally, while my mind
and creative imagination remain exploratory and wild. I often
wonder what forms of creative expression my mother might have
developed had she had the ample opportunities I enjoy. I am the
one who escaped but still carry what they call "survivor's guilt."

Like me, Mom loves words and word play. Creatively expres-
sive in ways all her own, she cultivates the bright shapes of
marigolds, arranging garden displays replete with leaping frogs
on whose eyes she fastens glittering sequins. She plays piano and
longs to be a bar lounge queen. When not tormented by fear,
she specializes in laughter and is a Buddha of compassion and
laughter to her friends. Everyone adores her; she is supremely
lovable, much more fun and less serious than her daughter. She
tells me to let go and not study so hard, to relax and eat more.
From the age of about twelve, I have been her elder in terms of
shouldering responsibility.

She remains, even in age, the playful one, the archetypal child,
the trickster fox. Strangely, both of us are Geminis, the sign of the
twins. I think of the words of Baudelaire: "—*Hypocrite lecteur,—
mon semblable,—mon frère!*" but modify the words: "*Cher maman,
ma semblable—ma soeur!*" After my father dies prematurely of ALS
(Lou Gehrig's Disease) and she moves into her final years, our sense
of closeness increases.

Thin and Unable to Swallow

You seem to be shrinking
in the big car he left you

with its crimson velour interior
and good sound system.

Your head barely crests
the top of the head rest
and you are still licensed
at 73; so you glide at 15 mph
in a 40-mile zone
ignoring the obscenities
of men buzzing past in fast cars.

At intersections you wait
till the traffic has cleared
for a mile in either direction
before venturing out.

Your body, that always
enveloped magnitude,
is now frail, and osteoporosis
slopes your shoulders.

It is strange to see you thin,
just as your mother
would have liked.
In your dreams she still
whispers, "Too bad hon,
you could have been a beauty
queen or a movie star."

You used to enjoy double-dip cones
but now you cannot swallow in public.

Dancing with Dementia

In her declining years in various care facilities the symptoms of
anxiety gradually fold into dementia, but what emerges unac-
countably is an inner calm, peace even, I had not witnessed before.

Once, while chatting with her on the phone, she pauses, speaks emphatically to proffer this lasting gift: "Susie, you are remarkable, a remarkable woman!!" I feel badly because just the day before I had complained to my husband that we ought to set up an "uh huh" machine to take her calls. As long as the "uh huhs" arrived at suitable intervals, she would never know the difference.

When visiting her in her final year, without catching my eye or acknowledging my presence in any other way, she begins referring to me in the kindest, most loving terms, speaking my name over and over.

During her last hours, I have the privilege of sitting with her for several hours in the home, holding her parchment hand. There is a Bible beside her bed so I pick it up and read from the place where it speaks of being "born again." If you want eternal life, the words say, you don't go back into your mother's womb again but through to another kind of birthing. In a place in the heart beyond belief, I feel somehow that what we call her mental illness, seen in another light, is part of an agonizing rebirth. A few weeks after her memorial service, my husband sees her in a dream sitting in a chair, swinging her legs over one side, laughing, and holding forth in conversation with a group of light-hearted friends. Who knows whether in a deeper place beyond our knowing this may not reflect the status of her soul.

Postscript

I remember your gesture
thrusting away open tins of spoiled food
your stories of the South, and jokes

soft-current speech
memory of inaccurate memory
antithetical to someone else's.

I cannot ask you for the facts
for what are facts to you
who would be annoyed by this

pestering of the past
this uneasy ahistoric chronicle,
tale told to hold what lineage

what line against chaos, for love
and the listening stars?

Dislocated Tongues

KEVIN SPENST

In February 2004, I began work on a one-act play about my schizo-phrenic father, a man who'd been largely absent through most of my life. I typed the first draft through three or four evenings in a loft my girlfriend and I had just moved into. I rolled my chair back from my desk and stretched my arms and hands, which were cramped from my new keyboard. My eyes closed and I tried to remember the sound of my father's voice. There was nothing but the clicking staccato heels of a neighbour upstairs.

Finally, I decided to call my mom.

"Just a second, let me adjust my hearing aid," she said.

She updated me on her busy schedule of carpet bowling, a Red Hat lady event, and shopping for the older people in her retirement community. At the ends of sentences her laughter chimed three notes up, and I turned our conversation to the play I was writing.

"I remember visiting Dad in Essondale, but I don't remember witnessing any of the craziness that landed him there." I knew of the time he'd gone to the airport to buy a one-way ticket to China, the time he bought a gun only to throw it in the Serpentine River for fear of what he'd brought into the home, the time he drove through a red light and smashed into another car after being on the move for forty-eight hours, and on and on. His life had been a trail of non sequiturs that I knew by heart.

"Oh he was off his rocker all right."

"But what did he do to get diagnosed as schizophrenic?"

"A week before your first sister was born, he locked himself in the bathroom and threatened to slit his wrists with a razor. The police and a doctor came over to sedate him and haul him off to Essondale. When your sister was born he was in the hospital."

I had to ask, "Why did you continue having kids?"

"We tried different birth controls, but they just didn't work and abortion wasn't an option. Sylvia was an IUD failure, Beverly was a rhythm method failure, and you, ten years later, you were a pill failure. We're glad we had you, and your sisters were happy to have a baby brother, but if your father had managed to fly to China that would have made raising all of you a lot easier."

"So we're a family of mistakes."

Her three-toned laugh pulled me into the present. My own aspirated laugh filled the large dimensions of the loft.

I rolled the chair back to the computer. The play would take months of rewrites. I was to perform it in September for the Vancouver Fringe Festival. The first scene involved an imaginary popcorn helmet, which I represented by plucking invisible kernels from my head. Ideas turned into something tangible at my fingertips.

It was going to be a crazy play about schizophrenia.

■ ■ ■

My first memory of my father was of him reading *The Wind in the Willows* to me at bedtime. He was still living at home, so I must have been about four. He read to me about Ratty and Mole drifting down a river and I stared, my mouth open, at the picture of fully clothed rodents in a blue rowboat, a silent scene more permanent than any words could conjure, although I could feel those words buzzing through my father's side. His two-hundred-odd pounds sunk him into my bed while I nestled into the warmth of his body.

Midway through the book, Pan made an appearance in order to remove the animals' memories of an unsettling incident "lest the awful remembrance should remain and grow, and overshadow mirth and pleasure." Perhaps my father read this line over my blond head to lull my memory from the turbulence behind our family. Or maybe he prayed that night for himself, as he tried to forget what had been almost twenty years in and out of Essondale with its treatments of electric-shock therapy and drugs. Maybe he prayed that my mother, who had taken him back so many times, would someday forget the evening he'd hung all his clothes outside on the lowest branches of two pine trees or the times he'd disappeared for days on end. Incomprehensible plots happening right over my head. My father's *mother*-tattooed arm squeezed me into his body before he kissed my forehead goodnight.

And then the light in the middle of the ceiling went out.

Several months after that night, my father invited Pan, Ratty, Mole, and the rest of the seen and unseen world into our home.

"Everyone's welcome in my house," he shouted to the street as he went from room to room opening windows. My mother closed them behind him, but he kept opening them again. Cold night air rushed into the house. He ran down the stairs to open the basement door along with more windows. Some shimmer of odd enthusiasm in his voice, or perhaps it was his eyes, triggered an alarm in my mother's head. She took me and my three sisters outside and into the car. We drove through the night to her parents' place in Abbotsford where we stayed for several days.

She went to a lawyer and got a restraining order placed on her husband and my father, Abram Spenst; he was to never set foot on our property again. From then on, after his releases from Essondale, he would have to fend for himself.

His recitation of *The Wind in the Willows* had worked: apart

from scraps of memory, the most dramatic event of my childhood—
my father's illness—was a big blank. Something I had to reconstruct
through questions over the phone with my mom.

■ ■ ■

"Take a break from the play," my girlfriend, Lisa, suggested. She
breathed in deep through almost fully closed lips. A sign of stress.
"Let's go out tonight."

She was right.

We walked to Tinseltown to watch a movie, *Evelyn*. At the beginning of the film, when the main character's father died, I fought back
tears. Lisa squeezed my hand. Countless times, she'd seen me tense
up and cry over the poorly acted death scenes of fathers in even
poorer movies. I tried to smile. She wiped the tears from my face with
the sleeve of the blue sweater I'd bought her for her birthday, and we
laughed at the ridiculousness of tears shed for a second-rate actor.

To breathe easy.

■ ■ ■

When I was about eight, the phone rang with the news that my
father was once again in Essondale. My mother put on her coat and
we got into the Buick to drive across the bridge. She turned off the
busy highway into the quiet entranceway. We drove up the narrow
road through a garden of trees and bushes. At the base of one tree,
a man sat in pyjamas as if he hadn't a care in the world. Farther up,
another man walked alone across the grass.

We parked in front of a large brick building. We walked up at
least one flight of stairs.

We stepped into a large, rectangular room. I saw my father staring out a window. There were other bodies in other chairs. There
were some men slowly shuffling across the floor, as if alone in a
field. My father sat slouched over.

My mom asked me to hug him. He barely moved under my
arms. Electric-shock therapy had answered his prayers.

■ ■ ■

"You know that 'Hello, my baby, hello, my honey, hello, my rag-time gal'? Or however that song goes."

The director of my play, an actor friend who'd been through several fringe festivals, nodded her enthusiastic, tilted smile.

"That's the tune I want to sing this part in."

She danced across the open space of the loft with exaggerated gestures while humming the ditty.

"Something like that?"

I re-read the lines and tried some of the moves out myself.

"He was my pappy, he was my father, he was my schizo dad. He was in the looney bin, there goes my memory of him. The gardens were gorgeous but brick buildings so scary, I didn't want to be left alone. Oh daddy, get sane soon, and teach me to ride a bike."

We spent the afternoon finding the footing for each word.

■　■　■

On Saturday afternoons, my Uncle Hans came with us to visit my father.

Uncle Hans always greeted me in a voice that soothed like a wooden wind instrument. "So, you ready to go?"

I nodded and we were on our way, this time to Scottsdale Mall, a trip exaggerated into hours in my nine-year-old head as we drove out beyond the familiar gas stations, houses, and the junk-shack convenience stores of the Fraser Highway. On the way, my uncle attempted to break through my silence. "Petro Canada, do you know what that stands for?" He chuckled. "Pierre Elliot Trudeau Ripped Off Canada." I had no notion of politics, a subject that my mother and three sisters never discussed, but I warmed to the thought of being included in some certainty of the adult world. Then, my uncle talked to me about my father. My mind drifted with the timbre of his voice.

When we arrived at the mall, my father was sitting on a bench just inside the front entrance. He saw me and resurrected a smile. As per the routine, I stepped into a bear hug that enveloped me in the sweat and smoke of his second-hand clothes. After my release, I looked around at the strangers shopping, wishing my father was one of them, remembering the time he had made a surprise appearance at my school. I'd had to leave class to go outside to talk to him by the hopscotch cross. My father struggled to find the right words to say while I glanced into the school to see if anyone was watching us.

In the mall, my uncle left us alone.

"I want to go to a toy store," I said, and we walked together until I sighted the Promised Land of Plastics. I raced in to gaze at a wall of *Star Wars* action figures. I picked a Boba Fett. $6.99. My father was unemployed, living on his monthly disability cheques, but he reached for his wallet, thick with notes, prescriptions, and individual photos of me and my three sisters. After he bought Boba Fett for me, I wanted to grab the toy from my father's hands and run to find a darkness to play under. I'd seen a therapist that summer near Guildford Mall who met with me and my sisters to assess our mental health and to explain to us our father's condition, the reasons why we'd spend our lives visiting him at a mental hospital. All I remembered of the visit was afterwards standing outside his office door with nothing in my hands. No reward for the vague discomfort associated with my father.

As we stepped out from the toy store, I tore off the plastic casing around Boba Fett. I put his blaster in his right hand, moulded for this singular purpose. My father sighed, put his hand on my shoulder, and said he was sorry. He said he loved me. I dreamt of other places and things in a galaxy far, far away.

■ ■ ■

I paced behind the black curtains as people shuffled into the theatre. The pre-show music, several of my girlfriend's original recordings on vocals and guitar, was quickly drowned out by the din of the audience. The lights dimmed and the crowd grew quiet.

I closed my eyes and ran through my lines alone:

And then I shrink down like Dennis Quaid in *Inner Space* and I'm soaring through brain cells, riding along synapses to understand my father's psychology from the inside. Flashing Rorschach inkblot cards in front of his brain cells, asking his neurons, "How does this one make you fire? How does this one make you fire?"

I heard my opening cue and walked onto the stage. For an hour, twenty-two characters and reams of absurdist lines rolled out of me. Each performance a ritual in therapy.

■   ■   ■

In the play of memory after memory, here is the hardest scene, which comes from when I was fourteen.

I remember holding the phone in a tight grip, my mouth hanging open over the receiver. I was sitting in a chair by the kitchen table, the three metre-corkscrew cord of the phone tangled around my feet.

"He was in his room alone. The owners of the house heard a crash and came downstairs. They called the ambulance. He's in Emergency at the Royal Columbian." My sister's voice wavered over unshed tears.

I put the phone down, walked into the living room, sat down on the La-Z-Boy that my father had once occupied through days of depression, and my fourteen-year-old body crumpled under tears. When my mom got home from her job at K-Mart, we drove out to New Westminster where we stood with my sisters and their husbands over his stroke-broken body. Some sun came in through the tall window, lighting an otherwise dark and empty room. I held the metal railing on the side of his bed and listened as he breathed hard beneath the beep of a life-support system.

The doctor said he wouldn't make it through the night.

My father held on for six more years, his body half paralyzed, containing an increasingly troubled mind. My sisters visited him every week. I visited once a month. The automatic doors into the intensive care unit opened to a world of people slouched over themselves in wheelchairs stalled en route to unknown destinations. Sometimes my father was among them. Usually, he was in his bed in his small room. My shame and grief were hidden by my not knowing what to say.

"Hi, Dad, how are you doing?" my sister said in a chipper voice.

"Good." His caved-in smile revealed a tongue, which rested on a stubbly upper lip. "Good I 'av my teef."

My sister handed him a plastic cup with his false teeth. He picked them up and plunked them into his mouth.

"Is that better?" my sister asked, ever attentive to his needs.

His false teeth only helped a little to clarify his slurred speech, which was pulled down at his lip by an invisible fishhook. My sister sometimes translated the questions he directed at me. At other times he talked about his day, sometimes conjuring up problems with the nurses. On good days, I understood half of what he said.

I sometimes tried to talk.

"I just got back from Europe," I told him sometime in May 1991. I wanted to entertain him then with my travels, stories that would go in a novel about my adventures abroad to be called *The Inevitable Lamb*, a story starting with a hike through the south of Crete. But my father's world was a single room of comforts or discomforts, and Europe held no relevance, even to his previous lives in Winnipeg, Abbotsford, Surrey, Vancouver, and New Westminster.

Besides, I'd never write a book called *The Inevitable Lamb*. I'd fill dozens of journals with false starts to stories that devolved into puzzle pieces to abstractions, as I tried to understand the differences between crazy and schizophrenic, as I wrote about everything except for my father there in the hospital speaking in tongues.

I wish I'd sent him postcards from Europe. I wish I'd thought to read him stories from his Bible. I wish I'd written down his last words, words that came a few days before Christmas 1991.

Belly Button

JANE FINLAY-YOUNG

My baby sister's newly knotted belly button: at three and three quarter years old that is my first memory. And inside that memory is the bedroom where she was born, the baby and the mother. The mother, who a few years later became violent and was arrested, diagnosed as paranoid schizophrenic, and put away.

But first there was the gentle October sunlight washing through the room where the baby had just been born, at home. The slant of clear light blurred the room, made it warm and close. There were the quiet wet sounds of the baby. There was the rustle of sheets as the mother adjusted herself against the pillows, brushed her damp hair back from her face. Perhaps my other younger sister was there, and the midwife or the doctor. Perhaps there was a rusty blood after-smell, the instruments still about: bits of red-soaked cloth, metal bowls, needle and thread. I don't remember.

I remember the baby, the light, and the vaguely washed-out presence of the mother . . . my mother. Perhaps she was sleeping. Or perhaps she was just as she always was—not there, not really, a vagueness in her eyes. An awayness that easily, unexplainably, could turn bright and fiery.

Someone, my father no doubt, was changing the baby's nappy, his tall, careful body bending over her, his long fingers reaching out to stroke her bald head. That's when I saw it: bloody and raw on her otherwise soft, pink belly. It pumped in and out with her breath as if it were alive, as if it were a tiny mouth, punched at, hurt.

Something was wrong with the baby.

I backed away, my small spine and the palms of my hands finding the wall. The October morning light, blue as the nearby sea, could not erase the shock, could not correct the damage. Something terrible had happened.

What's wrong with her? I probably asked. And my father would have laughed and tried to tease me back across the room toward the baby. She's sick, I might have said, and I would have released my palms from the wall momentarily to point at the sick place.

Or I might have asked, Who hurt her? And again he would have laughed, not a mocking laugh, just a laugh that was trying to be reassuring, a laugh that showed he loved curious questions and observations. He would have laughed and then explained, That's where she's been attached to Mummy.

■　■　■

We were not attached to Mummy. No, that's not true. We were fiercely attached. *She* was not attached to us. The more distant she became, the harder we clung. Until we couldn't. Until, one day, when we were six and four and two, she was gone and not once, so the story goes, did we ask for her.

She went to jail, we were told many years later, because she tried to kill a woman. She went to court. And then she went to Broadmoor, an institution in England for the criminally insane.

■　■　■

God told me to do it, my mother explained when I was twenty-four and newly married and my new husband and I had gone to England for our honeymoon. We stopped by to see her. By then my mother's mental illness was being managed, more or less, by drugs, and she had been released into the care of her parents.

We sat on a picnic blanket in her parents' front garden, overlooking the sea. It was a cool, early summer afternoon. Breezy. She passed us both a glass of orange juice and sat down beside us on the blanket and began to talk about why she tried to kill the woman.

I remember my mother's bleached blond hair lifting in the wind, her blue eyes bright and alert. Every feature of hers so definite: cheekbones, nose, the bony ridges around her eyes. I don't remember her enough to describe them in detail, but I remember they were prominent, they were real. There was no doubting her presence. This was my mother; that fact was as unreal as it was true.

I argued with God, I tried to turn back. But He made me. I understood why He wanted her dead, of course, the woman was evil, bad for her children.

The sea, just across the road, tossed blue-grey in the wind as we listened to her talk. Seagulls floated overhead. The orange juice so brilliant and cool in its tall glass. I shivered. *Bad for her children* . . . I could see that she had no idea that she had been bad for her own.

I set the juice down on the grass and tried to warm my hands. I didn't like juice, I never have, she'd given it to me without asking. She began her story without asking too. Without asking anything about either of us—How was the wedding? Where did you meet? How are your holidays?—she knew nothing and asked nothing. She hadn't been told about our wedding until after the fact. She didn't care.

She cared about her story, about telling it to us on the picnic blanket, on the grass, by the sea, the wind chopping at her crazy words, tossing them around, playing with them foolishly. Her parents, no doubt, had been told to stay inside, to not interfere.

I started stabbing her, she said calmly, seeming suddenly bored by the conversation, detached from it, *but I was stopped by a passer-by*.

She had a knife. Or was it a sharp wooden stake? Over the years I seem to have been told two different things. It was on the high street of a town in the south of England. I imagine my mother's face, expressionless, her strong tanned arms thrust toward . . .

It could have been me, or my sisters; I had felt and seen her simmering rage many times. It could have been my father, or my aunt or my grandmother. It could have been any of us, but instead it was a stranger she tried to kill.

God told her to do it; eighteen years later after incarceration and psycho-active drugs she still believed that, she still believed she'd done nothing wrong.

As I sat there listening my mind began to blur. Perhaps it was the undeniable fact of her physical-ness, how tangible she was there, just inches from me, how strong-looking, how touchable. Perhaps it was all the "what ifs" floating about me: what if she was okay, what if she could become my mother, the mother I craved. I no longer remember the specifics of my delusion, but the desire to have her all right, I remember the strength of that.

■ ■ ■

What did I think when I saw my sister's raw, terrifying belly? Did I think my mother had done it? Did I sense, even then, that my mother was capable of harming? And what does one do when one is three and three quarters and she suspects her mother might be dangerous? Already, before I saw my sister's belly button, the world must have felt dangerous to me. Already I must have felt how unsafe it was, or I don't think this belly button memory, with its attendant mystery and dread, would have stuck so close all these years.

The world is not safe; this is what children of the mentally ill learn. Anything could happen. A car could . . . a husband could . . . a child might . . . the house, the money in the bank, the pain in the breast, the lump in the neck. Be careful crossing the street, never let go of your child's hand, pay attention, pay closer and closer attention, have a Plan B, never let your guard down, never let go. Always be prepared to run, to shut down. Hold on. Let go. Never be certain. Never be proud. Never dream. Never have faith. The world will not unfold as it should. Never love. Not completely.

No doubt this list could be pages long, but you get the picture. You know, we all know, in small ways and big, about being small in a big, uncertain world, and then carrying that smallness with us on our backs into adulthood. We're all afraid, I suppose, to one degree or another.

I wonder if, for all her bravado, my mother was afraid and her mental illness was all in service of trying to break free of fear. Pushing to the edge and jumping. Jumping out of her 1960s house-wife life, past the limitations and control. Jumping out of her mind and into . . .

Silly thoughts. The woman was chemically imbalanced. The wacky chemicals made her hallucinate, made her delusional. They made her a disciple for God, an apostle. They made her selfish, uninterested in her children. Fearless and fearful and grander in her head than anyone could ever imagine. They made her wildly creative. An insomniac. They made her smoke too much, drink too much, spend too much. They made her altogether too much.

She listened to Mahler too loud as she painted into the sleepless night, under dull lamp light, trying to shine the light on her dark-ness. A sweet, thick sherry sitting beside the turps and oils. A tick of paint across her cheek.

■   ■   ■

That windy summer day on the picnic blanket by the sea I watched my mother and wanted to believe she was all right. Right in the head: sane. I wanted to believe she was a mother, my mother. I listened for an understandable explanation, a rationale. I watched her strong, handsome face and wanted the rest of the world to be wrong.

Are you crazy? my new husband exclaimed when I began to voice a budding feeling that perhaps, after all, she might be okay.

We were driving away from the sea, from her, twisting along the narrow lanes, the clouds overhead gathering, the evening coming on.

My husband's mind was neatly divided into black and white, right and wrong. It wasn't possible for him to see the complications, the twists and turns. A mother is always a mother, even when she can't be. A child is always a child, even when she isn't. A child always needs a mother, even though . . .

The hedgerows, lush and tangled, crowded in on us. The road narrowed. And narrowed.

Was I crazy? Would I become crazy? Would my sisters? Would my children?

■ ■ ■

I became a mother myself, at twenty-eight. A few days later my mother died.

One of my preoccupations when I was pregnant was keeping my mother from knowing I was going to have a child. A silly preoccupation; I'd seen her only a few times since I was six years old—the time after I was married being one of three times, I think. I was in Canada and she in England. We never called each other. Sometimes she wrote to me—disjointed letters on thin blue airmail paper, full of capitalized and underlined words. Words like LOVE and TRUTH and ABSOLUTE. Often I didn't open the letters, but I kept them until the last trimester of my pregnancy and then I threw them out.

I was afraid of her. I was afraid of her indifference. And her potential interest. I was afraid she'd appear on my doorstep and want to be my mother. And a grandmother to my child. I was afraid she might harm my child, just as she'd harmed my sisters and me— not in physical ways but in subterranean ways that are so hard to get at and expel. I imagined her picking up my baby and snapping its neck.

My son was born after a long labour, just as my sisters and I had been born. Cord severed and neatly knotted. And then, a few days later, without knowing that I'd given birth, my mother died. Suddenly, at fifty-two, of a cancer that had run so quickly through her that it was only after an autopsy was performed that anyone knew what was wrong.

I suppose that the cancer in her body reflected the chaos, the wild fire, that was her life. Unable to keep the chaos in her mind from invading her life, unable to sustain relationships or hold down a job, she was consumed. Like Joan of Arc in the fire.

Her name was actually Joan. She was so alone. I write that as a rhyme purposefully. It distances me from the fact of her aloneness and the aloneness that plagues the mentally ill. Stripped of her children and husband and career, stripped of her home and her dreams. Her identity. Her credibility. Her humanness. Stripped of all that and given a designation: paranoid schizophrenic.

■ ■ ■

I am almost fifty-two myself, the age my mother was when she died. I have a child, a husband, a career. I have dreams and friends and family. I have a home. I have only fleeting memories of my mother, small shards that will never make up a whole. The way a room became compressed when she pushed into it. The light catching her blue, blue eyes. Her muscular calves. The sound of her nyloned legs scratching and rubbing together as she walked too fast to keep up with. The high-frequency buzz about her. Her eyes that never rested, at least not on me. Her leather skirts. Her bags full of make-up. Her high heels. Her sour odour. Her cigarillos. The snap of her lighted match. The dark and definite lines around the objects she painted. The distance that drew her forward. The heavens that pulled at her. The emptiness between her and the rest of us that day when I was three and three-quarters and she had just given birth to another child she would not be able to care for.

Family Constellation

One Girl in the Crowd

BETH ROWNTREE

I was born with childhood schizophrenia. What must or must not be behind my schizophrenia puzzles me to this day!!!

Actually my schizophrenia was diagnosed at two and a half years of age. I still have to take medicine from time to time, but I can get along fine without having to take so many pills and injections

I am very proud to be a full-blooded Canadian. I am a Rosenyarkatchian Eskimo with a little bit of Kutchin and Ukrainian in my ancestry. I was adopted in the family way and my older sister, Lenore, as a mixture of Rosenyarkatchian, Kutchin, and Ukrainian, was adopted herself.

I took a walk earlier in the day and thought if everyone in the world were like me in looks, etcetera—the world would be very funny indeed!

Often I sit by the fireside watching the flickering flames and wishing I had more to give and offer the world!

Yes it is true I have always enjoyed doing silk-screening especially the silk-screening that involves hard strenuous work not simple easy work. And I take the shortest passages and longest writing of all Bibles and other books literally, and I mean literally.

I am going to go shopping with Mom to buy some Christmas presents and look at the fancy decorated elves, Santa Claus, and reindeers. I can picture my sister, Lenore, as being the Princess Rose, and me as being the other Princess Rose, feeding the very special gifted reindeers loaded with small gifts of love.

There are billions of things I wish I could change about the world and one is everyone's outlook toward themselves.

Someday I hope to be the greatest silk-screening artist in the world!

I always got high marks in spelling, English, and all other subjects and character record, but more often than not I got very low marks especially in Mathematics, but not so much in clear thinking, reliability, health, thrift, and social attitude.

The subjects I like the best are fun and happiness!!!

There are times where I get a little bit too self-centred, sensitive, and touchy, and the rest of the world sometimes gets a little bit too wrapped up in themselves. I must write far too sensitive, far too touchy, and far too self-centred. And that goes for all the rest of us!

I thought I have lots of things going for me, a good home, good health, and two cats, Grinny and Tooney, whom I can turn to when I feel down not up about the world!

I thought I have a good home to come from. So if group homes, etcetera, fire me it's not the end of the world, but if I was kicked out of my real home I would never be able to stand the harsh reality and I might add frightening reality.

I thought I am in very good health physically, emotionally, and mentally. I have everything going for me, everything worth living for, everything to be thankful for plus a lot to offer the world!!!

I have always had things far too easy, not as gruesome as the rest of the world, and my parents aren't in the least bit strict or domineering compared to lots of other parents.

My mom is looking at the television guide, putting herself in neutral, as she always says, "Put yourself in neutral," to me. "You can't change the future. Wishful thinking will not make things happen."

It's time to take my uppers and read the *Observer* and the *Upper Room*, especially the *Upper Room* that makes jokes on religion not those dummy *Upper Rooms* that delve so literally into the real long writings of the Bible. They must be the disk for the Lord's slop!

A little bit of the sacramental wine!

I picture a sloppy-joe hamburger on top of Lenore's head cracking all sorts of jokes on religion. The funny thing is that I'm the sloppy-joe hamburger who always bugs my kid sister!

There are all sorts of me. First I'm the happy sort. Then I'm the sad sort and on down the yellow brick road!

My favourite poem is *If*.

My mom who is a kooky scientist says I need a lot more vitamins, protein, calcium, iron, and far less carbohydrates and no caffeine and alcohol!!!

I am having a mug of tea thinking that there are billions of things I must change about myself, and one is myself!

The schizophrenic lives in many different worlds, all private worlds of their own!

Like I do!

Yes it's true I do come out with a lot of fantasies, but I try to keep my fantasies to myself and not bother the world with my fantasies!!

I always enjoy writing short stories of princesses and dashing young handsome princes!! Especially princes with dark brown soft melting eyes!!! A lot of my short stories have sad endings not happy endings!!! But a lot of my short stories have happy ever after endings!!!

Yes I have been in a variety of rehabilitation centres, sheltered workshops, employment training centres, and schools, especially schools with opportunity classes. I don't know where I'll live, eat, and work once my family and all my friends pass away.

And I might add play!!!

If anyone has the understanding and patience for me then it's a real miracle!!! One thing I hope any places I go to work in or any places I live in in the far distant future will serve only home-cooked meals, especially Canadian meals like my mom makes!!!

Yes, world, in this autobiography I am writing I have tried extra hard to avoid nonsense, fantasies, lies, wrong impressions, lists, philosophizing, obviousness, generalities, well I won't go on, world!!!

One perfect example I follow is this one!

Say what you feel!!!
Write what you feel!!!!
Do what you feel!!!

Wear what you feel!!!
Go where you feel!!!
Send what you feel!!!
Edit what you feel!!!
Omit what you feel!!!
BELIEVE what you feel!!!

Another perfect example I follow is less talk more action!

Actions speak louder than words!!!

I don't know what brought on my childhood schizophrenia because it certainly wasn't alcohol, a bad home life, overprotection of myself, or anything that someone blood-related or married-related did.

If there are any miracle cures or miracle healings for schizophrenia please, pretty please, let me know, friends!!!

Faith, man, machines, tests, examinations, informations, etcetera, won't do a single darn thing for me unless I help myself!

If there are any courses, etcetera, you would love me or like me to join, enter, support, or get really involved in, then please, pretty please, let me know, family and friends.

Someday I would love to be an embroiderer and embroider all sorts of skating costumes and especially pictures of beauteous scenery.

At a rough estimate I would estimate that my writing at its very best would gross a dollar a piece and my embroidery would sell for a dollar a piece!!! When it comes to embroidery I would specialize in both beaded and crewel!! My writing would specialize in fiction and non-fiction books especially ones having to do with crafts and needlework that people really go for!!!

Christmas at our home is a family social affair. My mom prepares a Christmas Eve supper. Where the Christmas Eve supper will come from this year I don't know. But I hope the Christmas Eve supper will come from Dreamamania, my magical land for gnomes that always go about fantasizing and dreaming, plus wishful thinking like me!!!

What my chemical imbalance is I don't know but I sure am curious. If I knew what my chemical imbalance was then I would be able to seek out new miracle drugs to get me cured.

I put faith in medical healing, therapeutic healing, spiritual healing, faith healing, and love healing plus many other curings and healings all having to do with herbal teas, friends.

There's one thing that's good about my dad, he always thinks more of the world than himself!!!

Yes, Santa Claus, I would like a book on writing especially one that deals with autobiographies and biographies.

If anyone would like to omit or edit from my autobiography, because I plan to edit and omit a lot, please let me know.

I remember going to the Exhibition when it was first opened and begging my parents to let me go on the rides. When I could not go on the rides I liked the best, like the Ferris wheel, then I felt very disappointed and somewhat upset.

I also remember Grandma's last words to me—"Get me a pillow, Bethey."

I would like to continue on writing this autobiography but I am tired.

My Life as Beth

My I go on!
A conversation with God
Small Christmases
Winnie the Pooh Bible
Cosmetic's Bible
The Holy Bible scanned
Horses, and that has nothing to do with me riding
horses,
Elvis Presley's Private Party
A Hard Day's Night
Breathtaking
One Girl in the Crowd
I call myself Beth
Embroidery, and that has nothing to do with me
embroidering,
My I go on with interests!
Interest, interest, interests, and that has nothing to do
with me taking a genuine interest,
My I go on with that!
Avoid fuck when I don't always avoid lies,
sins, dishonests, insinceres, nonsenses, non sequiturs,
Knitting, and that has nothing to do with me knitting,
My I go on with my voice!
My truths, my insinceres, my loyalties, my directs, my
straightforwards,
the Spanish lace gown, the Ukrainian lace gown,
peace and war,
war and peace, the Irish lace gown,
My I go on, but tell lies!
Batiking, and that has nothing to do with me batiking,
Silk screening, and that has nothing to do with me
silk screening,

I go on with knit one, knit two and that's boring.
I go on to all kinds of embroidery stitches and that has nothing to do
with being silent or quiet on embroidery, satin stitches, pretty eye stitches,
the silent stitch, the silent partner, silent justice, silent honour, correct sex,
experiencing sex with a man and a boy.
Happy to keep silent for seconds
Happy to keep silent for moments
Happy to keep silent for hours
Happy to keep silent for years
Happy to keep silent for decades
Happy to keep silent for centuries
My I go on to a voice, to truths, sinceres, loyals, directs, and straight forwards.
And right now I am lost in a real world and an unreal world!!!
Right now I am thinking of Kay!!!
Thinking of Jill!!!
Julie building her castles.
I shed a tear for every schizophrenic victim, for every schizoid victim.
I am a happy victim with my silent voice box, silent voice box strings.

Flat Champagne

LENORE ROWNTREE

It's a Saturday night in the autumn of 1960, long enough after supper that there's no chance my mother is going to issue a last-minute bathtub order. In fact, I'm golden to stay up for at least another hour because nothing is going to get her off the couch before the champagne bubble world of *Lawrence Welk* comes to its usual accordion and fiddle, or accordion and clarinet, or accordion and some other silly instrument, mashed-up ending.

My father, a jazz musician, is downtown at a club on Yonge Street. My baby sister is asleep in her crib. And my younger sister, Beth, is somewhere in the house—defacing a Bible, a dictionary, or one of our precious picture books. I'm nine and Beth is eight, and we're both attached to the picture books, both still think they are ours to do with as we want, even though they were our father's first. I've tried to put *Chicken Little* and *Grasshopper Green* out of harm's way, but when Beth finds the books, she writes things in them like *I'm afraid, I want my mommy!* In the back of A.A. Milne's *When We Were Very Young*, she's written our address, but she's misspelled the street—it says we live at *11 Horror Hill*—and she's printed our phone number with all the figures backwards. Beth will write on anything she can get her hands on, and she never seems to stop talking. Increasingly her talking, sometimes shouting, is about things that don't make any sense.

And me, well, I'm sitting at our pull-down kitchen table where I spend a lot of time dreaming about things. On Saturday nights, I'm usually dreaming about being Janet Lennon, the youngest of the four sisters from Venice, California, who sing their hearts out every week for Lawrence Welk. When I hear them being introduced, I leave my post at the table and stand at the top of the stairs where I can see the TV. But I don't go down to the den to sit beside my mother because what I really want is to get back to the table as soon as the song ends, to play with my Lennon Sisters Cut-Out Dolls.

The dolls are made of cardboard punched out of the first page of the book. To me, they are beautiful. I line them up on the table and admire their sparkling hair and perfect makeup. Each sister has a wardrobe I cut from the book using a sharp pair of nail scissors, carefully guiding the point around the pleats, frills, and cuffs, always careful not to cut off any of the tabs. I need the tabs to fold the edges of the clothing over onto the dolls. The shoes are tricky, especially around the heels, but the toughest to cut out is the gorgeous lemon yellow swing coat that belongs to Janet. Every time I play with Janet something deliciously Lennon-sister-lemon-pie-happy swims through my mind.

I love playing where pleasure laps at the shores of beauty, fame, and talent without letting myself get too specific about what I am doing. Because getting specific means admitting I'm escaping a distressed mother tuning out with Lawrence, and an unwell sister scribbling and muttering in the basement. So I sit in the relative quiet of our after-supper kitchen, the air still full with the pungent smell of the spaghetti we've wolfed down, and I trace my scissors around the silks, brocades, and embroideries of a perfect life, careful to cut around the difficult edges, the unexpected corners, vigilant not to cut off the life-linking tabs. When everything is ordered and cut perfectly, I can forget that even the lemon-chiffon swing heaven of Janet's coat could be destroyed. It is after all just a piece of paper, like any other, and it can be written on, made to hold a list of bizarre and forlorn words.

And the worst of it is that I am playing with sister dolls instead of with my own sister who just a year or two before was my best friend.

■　■　■

There is a scene I replay in my mind. We are at the cottage and a gang of us is pulling away from the dock in one of the boats. Either it is our plywood runabout with its noisy 3 hp Evinrude or it is the Chapple kids' rowboat named *Cinq* for the five of them and for the auditory pun. It's odd because in the replay there's no noise except for my father calling, yet we pull away with some authority, which makes me think we are under power. We are going somewhere to which Beth has not been invited. She is standing on the dock with her orange lifejacket and Dad is saying, *Take Beth with you.*

Dad looks sad, Beth looks sad. We do not come back. Situations like this make him ask me, *Would you kick a cripple?* His logic is simple, and evidently, yes, I would kick a cripple.

■　■　■

By early adolescence Beth has a full-blown writing obsession. She still underlines words in the dictionary and ticks sad words in the Bible, but she's gone beyond that. None of the pens or pencils in the house work, they're either dry or broken. No piece of paper is safe from complete obliteration. She is no longer able to go to school because there is no school where it is safe for her to go. The education system doesn't yet have any of the concepts of integration and acceptance. The troubled kids, whether they be juvenile delinquents, young addicts, sexually promiscuous, or mentally ill, all end up at the same vocational school where they can do maximum harm to one another and receive little specialized help.

Beth looks like a confused visitor in most of the family photos: the Christmas gift frenzy, the Halloween spectacle, photos even of

her own birthday party. The camera captures an image of someone
brought in to observe the traditions of a group of humans who are
not wired the same way as she. Her idea of getting organized is to
write lists:

Experience Thoughts
Funk and Wagnall Thoughts
Excited Thoughts
Lord Thoughts
Almighty Thoughts
Miracle Worker Thoughts
Jesus Thoughts
Patronized Saints Thoughts
Canonized Thoughts
Open Minded Thoughts
Giggling Thoughts
Laughing Thoughts
Needing Thoughts

The list reads like a type of want ad: *Seeking Normal Thoughts*.
And it's born in the mind of someone who has schizophrenia, or
autism, or brain damage at birth, or some other unknown genetic
predisposition to madness. The experts are all over the map, and I
am terrified when they come to the house to take our fingerprints.
Terrified they will find I have the same *crazy* whorl. I watch to see
if their eyes light up or gleam in a different way after they look at
mine. But then no one ever gets back to us because nothing is con-
clusive and the professionals don't like uncertainty, and my mother
withdraws into further lockdown because the current trendy theory
is that schizophrenia is born in generations of bad mothering. And
all of it is insensitive and dehumanizing and leads me to be suspicious of the medical profession, who spend a lot of time talking
about the tragic disease my sister has, as if we are all watching a car
wreck on television involving no one we know.

Every day Beth fills hundreds of pages with her lists, a type of mad slam poetry. She can't organize her thoughts but she can organize her lists. I get through high school by pretending I belong to another family and trying to ignore what goes on at our house.

■ ■ ■

Three things happen in the summer of 1969 that have an unlikely but dramatic impact on me. First, William Lennon, father of the Lennon Sisters, is killed by a delusional fan who believes William stands in the way of his marriage to sister Peggy. Then, Charles Manson and his ragtag family, composed primarily of girls not much older than myself, go on their Helter Skelter rampage. Finally, Neil Armstrong becomes the first human to set foot on the moon. All of this makes a spicy stew in my head. I learn that shitty things happen to nice people, shitty things happen to famous people, and there really are no limits to time, space, or whatever can happen in the universe.

I am a university dropout working as a bank teller in the day and lying in bed at night not sleeping. Like most eighteen-year-olds I have big questions in my mind, but I'm not too sure how many others' questions go anything like this: *Should I kill myself because I've had random thoughts that my sister and my family would be better off if she were dead, so therefore I am no better than that deranged creep Charles Manson—I, too, am a murderer—and for that I should be put to death or at least locked up, and since I don't have the guts to kill myself, should I do something horrible and stupid like Manson to get myself locked up, or should I join a convent and let the nuns figure me out, but since I'm not Catholic should I just go ahead and kill myself now?*

I start searching in earnest for that crazy fingerprint whorl of mine.

■ ■ ■

By the mid-1980s, Beth is in her thirties and still living at home where she's left alone to rant most days because no one can take being with her for long—it has become her *Horror Hill*. When I look into her face I can see even she can't stand to be with herself anymore. She's become a disappointed member of the 999 Queen Street West asylum crowd in downtown Toronto. She visits a psychiatrist regularly on the tenth floor of the Clarke Institute of Psychiatry. Intermittently, she's lived unsuccessfully in two different group homes, one of which was across from the 100 Huntley Street headquarters where the spectre of religious salvation became a fascination for her, and in both of which she's been sexually assaulted. And it's very hard to say exactly whose fault any of this is.

But by December 1984, I figure I've grown up, I've gone to law school, I'm going to be able to figure this out. Except what am I really doing? I'm dropping in for the requisite five-day Christmas visit with family, I'm circling around Beth like I'm still getting used to the idea of her being related to me. And I'm holding out a three-ring binder saying, *Here, unravel it yourself—tell your own life story.* So she does. She writes an autobiography entitled *One Girl in the Crowd* and she starts it with the simple admission, *I was born with childhood schizophrenia. What must or must not be behind my schizophrenia puzzles me to this day!!!*

She has a much clearer view of it than I. I can't even look her in the eye without dissolving. I retreat back to Vancouver where I have moved to get away from it all, but I don't really get away. She is inside me like a grain of sand in my heart.

■ ■ ■

Years later, I am home again for the holidays and the family has driven to the group home where Beth lives north of the city. She tries her best with her appearance, but she is often clothed in smelly sweatpants and a stained T-shirt. The staff at the home is over-worked, and Beth no longer has the skills to take proper care of her hygiene. She has developed an unnatural fear of hot water and frequently tells us about the resident who made a bath with scalding water and suffered a fatal heart attack. I don't know how much of the event is relayed accurately, but the impact is real enough.

Beth shuffles down the icy path of the home toward the car. She is carrying her tattered black vinyl purse. I look inside the purse and find nothing in it but scraps of paper so covered in writing there is hardly any white left on the pages. When we get home, I take the contents from the purse and put them in a Ziploc bag. I am treating the rubble like a museum artifact, trying to distance myself from its sadness. I still have the contents, in the bag, together with the card she gave me that year. It says, *I'm so glad you are here with me at Christmas.* She's resisted writing anything more on the card except the words *with the best of my love.*

■ ■ ■

There is something I knew when I was young that took me almost fifty years to get back. After years of struggling, and mental health warehousing for Beth, she has moved to a group home near me in Vancouver. One day, we are in her bedroom at the new home and David Bowie's "Let's Dance" comes on the radio. As we sometimes used to do, we start to dance.

She's the one with schizophrenia, but I'm the one who's lived my life in a delusion, a dream that I bring respect and non-judgment to her. When I deal with Beth, there is no artifice from her, I'm dealing with her where she's at—no amount of cajoling, manipulating, or bribing will put her into another state, another need, another moment. But when she is dealing with me, she is working with a manipulator, a con artist, someone who too many times has put up a front of compassion and caring while secretly thinking this is too hard, she is too smelly, too difficult to be around. But on this day, she has on her blue eye shadow and her baby pink lipstick, she's had a bath, and we're dancing. Out of nowhere I tell her, *You're my best friend.* She just looks at me and says, *I know.* For the moment all her wiring is intact and I know that she knows.

I didn't even realize how much of the friendship I'd lost until it came back. To love someone who is complicated requires you not to think too deeply sometimes, to simply put on your party makeup and dance.

Afterword
ANDREW BODEN

Many of the essays in this collection have been about troubling events in the lives of ordinary, caring people. I consider myself an ordinary, caring person, but at times I fear my normality conceals a disturbing dynamic. Early on in my brother's mental illness, his friends deserted him. This is a common response to people with mental illness and one I've struggled to control in myself for twenty years, to fight my fear, disgust, and frustration. Those who suffer psychotic reactions may not only suffer the isolation of friendlessness but also commitment to a mental hospital. I saw few visitors in the Sherbrooke Centre, the psychiatric facility at the Royal Columbian Hospital. For some, the ultimate segregation is homelessness, an appalling fate for too many people with mental illness in our era of closing mental institutions and choosing to underfund community supports.

Our desire to withdraw from people with mental illness has many sources, only one of which I want to mention here. I remember in my first psychology course our professor told us not to diagnose ourselves during the "abnormal psychology" section. That in the case histories of psychoses, we would see ourselves and begin to worry about our own sanity. Our professor tacitly acknowledged that the difference between a psychotic state and a normal one is in degree and not in kind. My so-called ordinary flaws exist on a continuum with psychotic ones: the psychotic being, as Gordon Claridge argues in *Origins of Mental Illness*, abnormal manifestations of flaws I already possess.

Author Marjory A. Bancroft wrote in her article "Nasrudin Looks at Mental Illness" that we should conceive of people with mental illness not as case histories but as symbols, as "[m]irrors, surely: the circus distorting-mirrors that exaggerate our every flaw." The point isn't to see our ordinary paranoias, vanities, and delusions as psychotic symptoms ("we're all psychotic") but to see our flaws at all, perhaps for the first time. I once suffered a psychotic reaction to the prescription antidepressant Remeron. When I recovered, I realized that my psychotic fantasy was my own vanity and egocentricity writ large. I could see their tyranny over my thoughts and decisions in a way I couldn't before my own psychosis; I could rally an inner resistance.

We can shrink away from a mirror or put it away so we never have to suffer its reflected light or we can come closer and look for a time—at ourselves.

Notes on Contributors

Andrew Boden's articles on mental illness have appeared in *Open Minds Quarterly* and *Other Voices*. His short stories and essays have been published in *The Journey Prize Stories 22, Geist, The New Quarterly, Prairie Fire, Vancouver Review*, and *Descant*. His story "The Parts of Ourselves Without Names" was a recent honourable mention in Glimmer Train Press's Family Matters fiction contest. He writes about his brother's schizophrenia. Please visit andrewboden.ca.

Dell Catherall lives in Vancouver, British Columbia, and is a retired teacher-librarian. Her short stories have won first place in *The Ubyssey's* literary contest and have been shortlisted for the *Vancouver Courier's* writing contest. Her poem "Witch Hazel (For a bi-polar son)" appeared in *Arborealis: A Canadian Anthology of Poetry 2010*. She began taking creative writing courses to help her deal with the many issues her family faced after her son's diagnosis with bipolar disorder.

Jennifer Crowder worked for seventeen years at a Seattle corporation before leaving to write creative non-fiction. She has completed certificate programs in writing memoir and literary non-fiction through the University of Washington Extension. She holds degrees in English from the University of North Carolina at Chapel Hill and Scripps College in Claremont, California. One of her essays appears in *We Came to Say*, a collection of memoir written by students of Theo Nestor at the UW and edited by Theo. Jennifer is currently at work on a memoir. She writes about the life lessons she continues to learn from her uncle, who struggles with schizophrenia.

Meredith Darling is a graduate of the Professional Theatre Program of Dawson College in Montreal, Canada (The Dome Theatre). A version of this story was produced for the 1999 Montreal Fringe Theatre Festival as the play *Garden of Edie*. Her recent work can be found in anthologies, including *Delicious* and *Leonard Cohen: You're Our Man*, and magazines such as *The Toronto Quarterly*. She writes about a difficult period when she was hospitalized with schizophrenia.

Sara Demeter is a poet, novelist, and teacher.

Jane Finlay-Young published her first novel, *From Bruised Fell*, with Penguin in 2000. She has also published short stories in literary magazines; contributed a non-fiction piece to the anthology *The First Man in My Life* (Penguin, 2007); and co-published *Watermelon Syrup* (WLU, 2007), a novel Jane revised for Annie Jacobsen after her death. Jane has just completed a memoir, *Certain*, about her foray into Orthodox Judaism. She lives in Halifax. She writes about growing apart from a mother who suffered from schizophrenia.

Yaho-Hanan Fiwchuk was born Nicholas John Fiwchuk. After a twenty-year hiatus from art, he has been painting feverishly since 2007 and has shown at various locations around Vancouver, including the Gallery Gachet and the Havana Gallery. As well, he is part of the Art Studio's Travelling Show, and he is especially happy about his very successful showings each year at the Art Studio Winter Sale. His tale is one of recovering over and over again from schizophrenia.

Clarissa Hart is a graphic artist who lives in California and contributes her comic about her experiences with PTSD. When not doodling, Clarissa enjoys podcasts, historical trivia and is hoping for an end to California's drought.

Laura Ingram is a tiny girl with large glasses. She lives in Virginia and writes in this collection about her experiences with anorexia. Her poetry and prose have also been published in *Five on the Fifth, If and Only If, Gravel* magazine, *The Cactus Heart Review, Noise Medium, Tallow Eider Quarterly, Forest for the Trees, Teenage Wasteland, Sugar Rascals*, and over a dozen other magazines and journals. Laura works as a contributing writer for The Odyssey Online. She writes fiction and poetry about anything and everything, and enjoys most books and all cats.

Jamie Johnson's full-length memoir *Secret Selves* won an IPPY award in the Best Regional Non-Fiction category for Eastern Canada. Her memoir takes the reader through the most difficult years of her two children's lives—one who transitioned from female to male, the other who shared his body with five alternate personalities. It is a book of hope for struggling parents. Jamie has been published in the *Globe and Mail, True North Perspective, Homemakers Magazine*, and in a resource book called *Families in TRANSition*. She lives with her husband in Ontario, Canada.

Fiona Tinwei Lam is a Vancouver-based writer born in Scotland and the author of two books of poetry, *Intimate Distances* (Nightwood, 2002), which was a finalist for the City of Vancouver Book Prize, and *Enter the Chrysanthemum* (Caitlin, 2009). She is a co-editor of and contributor to the non-fiction anthology *Double Lives: Writing and Motherhood* (McGill-Queens, 2008). Her work has been published in literary magazines Canada-wide, broadcast on CBC, and appeared in more than sixteen anthologies, including *The Best Canadian Poetry 2010* (Tightrope Books). The poem "Aftermath" from *Intimate Distances* has been reprinted in this book with permission from the publisher and will resonate with anyone who has had experiences with hospitalization.

Erin Hart MacNair is a freelance writer, mother, and metalsmith. She's been published in the *BC Council for Families Newsletter*, *blush magazine*, *Reality Mom*, the *Globe and Mail*, and placed second in the 2010 annual Memoirsink.com writing contest. Her online links can be read at erinmacnair.com. Erin lives in Vancouver, BC, with her family and her ancient cat. She misses her father, who committed suicide in the face of his fight with what was then called manic depression.

Born in Budapest, **Gabor Maté**, MD, immigrated to Canada at the age of twelve. He spent some time working as a teacher before returning to university to pursue his lifelong dream of becoming a doctor. He ran a popular family practice for many years, and spent twelve years working in Vancouver's Downtown Eastside, caring for patients suffering from mental illness, drug addiction, and HIV. In the 1990s, Dr. Maté was a regular medical columnist for the *Vancouver Sun* and the *Globe and Mail*. He is also the author of four works of non-fiction. His book, *In the Realm of Hungry Ghosts: Close Encounters With Addiction*, won a Hubert Evans Award in 2010. In addition to being a physician and bestselling author, Dr. Maté is a highly sought-after public speaker. He has three grown children and currently resides in Vancouver, BC, with his wife. Please visit drgabormate.com.

Susan McCaslin is an established Canadian poet, faculty emeritus of Douglas College in Westminster, British Columbia, and author of eleven volumes of poetry, including her most recent, *Demeter Goes Skydiving* (University of Alberta Press, 2011). The volume has been nominated for a BC Book Prize (Dorothy Livesay Poetry Prize) and an Alberta Book Publishing Award (Robert Kroetsch Poetry Book Award). Susan has also published a new volume of essays, *Arousing the Spirit: Provocative Writings* (Wood Lake Books, 2011). She has edited two anthologies of spiritual poetry and is on the editorial board of *Event: the Douglas College*

Review. She writes about her mother's struggles with an affliction that may have begun as bipolar disorder but was diagnosed as schizophrenia in 1963. Her mother's paranoiac delusions were possibly triggered by the diet medication she was prescribed in the 1960s. Susan lives in Fort Langley and Victoria, BC. Please visit susanmccaslin.ca.

Judy McFarlane graduated with an MFA in creative writing from UBC in 2005. Her work has been published in the *Vancouver Sun*, the *Globe and Mail*, a BC Federation of Writers' anthology, and *Room*, where her short story "Pill-Sorting for Dummies" placed in the 2010 fiction contest and was later nominated for the Journey Prize. Her essay "On the Way to Here" placed in the BC Federation of Writers' 2010 non-fiction contest. She produced *Amazing Grace* and *I Live on Fraser Street* for CBC radio. Judy's brother was diagnosed in his late fifties with bipolar disorder.

Lauren McGuire is working on a memoir, *The Keeper of Secret Sorrows*, about her brother's battle with schizophrenia. She has previously published an article about her brother in *No Touching*, an American creative non-fiction magazine. She lives in Seattle, Washington, with her husband and two children.

Nicole Melchionda is a recent graduate of Stetson University in Florida. There she completed an independent study on gothic poetry with award-winning poet Terri Witek and worked closely with journalist Andy Dehnart. Her senior thesis explored how depression infiltrates a writer's work, which inspired her to examine her own experiences with the illness. She contributes her essay as an impassioned voice seeking to remove the stigmas that come with mental illnesses. Her poetry and essays have been featured in several presses such as *Helios Quarterly Magazine*, *Crab Fat* magazine, *Points in Case*, and *Red Dashboard Press*. When she's not writing, she's probably reading or watching videos of funny animals.

Shane Neilson is the author of several books of poetry, including *Alden Nowlan and Illness* (Frog Hollow Press, 2005), *Exterminate My Heart* (Frog Hollow Press, 2008), *Meniscus* (Biblioasis, 2009), and *Complete Physical* (The Porcupine's Quill, 2010). His essay "Elm" received an honourable mention in *Prairie Fire* magazine's 2007 creative non-fiction contest. He practises medicine in Erin, Ontario. He writes about a suicide attempt arising from depression and the role that poetry plays in his life.

Catherine Owen is a Vancouver writer. A former teen parent of two children, she went on to obtain her master's degree in English from SFU (Burnaby 2001) and to publish nine trade collections of poetry, her latest titled *Seeing Lessons* (Wolsak & Wynn, 2009). Her seventh title, *Frenzy* (Anvil Press), won the Alberta Literary Award for 2009. She also has a volume of essays and memoirs called *Catalysts: confrontations with the muse* (Wolsak & Wynn, 2012). Her essays have been published in *Subterrain* and in the online US journal *Radius*, in an anthology on Joe Rosenblatt, and in a collection titled *Double Lives: Essays on Writing and Mothering*. She writes about obsessive compulsive disorder in her family.

Andrea Paquette is a "bipolar babe" who has an inspiring story. She is dedicated to "stigma stomping" and shares her personal story in the community and in secondary and post-secondary classrooms. She's appeared in local and national media on a number of occasions, discussing her work as a mental health educator and showcasing the very successful Bipolar Babe Benefit: Hair Show and Art Gala. She has worked in the BC government in the areas of mental health, social development, and education, and she is the executive director of the Bipolar Disorder Society of British Columbia. The Bipolar Babe project website is bipolarbabe.com.

Addy S. Parker is currently working on her memoir, *Corporate Madness*, about her experiences as a bipolar corporate manager during the Silicon Valley tech boom.

Beth Rowntree is a compulsive writer; if she had her way, she would never stop writing. Her writing has been published in *The Unacknowledged Source* and *Geist*, and her poetry is included in the anthology *Best Canadian Poetry 2010* (Tightrope Books). The essay "One Girl in the Crowd" is a part of an autobiography she wrote in 1984 about her challenges with schizophrenia, and the poem "My Life as Beth" was written in 2009.

Lenore Rowntree's short stories and poetry have been published in several Canadian literary journals, and her poetry is included in the anthology *Best Canadian Poetry 2010* (Tightrope Books). Her play *The Woods at Tender Creek* was produced in Vancouver at the Cultch. Most recently her collection of short stories *Dovetail Joint* was published in 2015 by Quadra Books, and her novel *Cluck* was published in 2016 by Thistledown Press. She was shortlisted for a CBC Literary Award for the essay "Flat Champagne" written about her sister's childhood schizophrenia, featured in this collection. Her website is lenorerowntree.com.

Jill Sadowsky is a published South African author living in Israel, where she is an English tutor. The account of her son's suicide *Weep for Them* was published in Hebrew and sold more than eight thousand copies. Her book entitled *David's Story* has been posted on the Amazon Kindle Store. She has also published in numerous journals dealing with mental health and psychiatric issues, including the *Schizophrenia Bulletin*, *Horizons: The Jewish Family Journal*, the *Israel Journal of Psychiatry and Related Sciences*, and the *Greek Journal of Medical Services*.

Gail Marlene Schwartz is a writer and performer living in Montreal. Recently, her articles have appeared in *Parents Canada*, *GO Magazine*, and *Gay Parent*. She has toured her autobiographical solo play, *Crazy: One Woman's Search for Sanity*, to theaters and community venues across North America over the past four years. Her article about the play's development process, "Acting Crazy: Spying on, Jamming with and Crooning about Anxiety and Depression," was published by the Community Arts Network in October of 2009. Visit her blog, twodykesandaboyby.blogspot.com, and her company website, thirdstorywindow.com.

Kevin Spenst's fiction has appeared in the anthology *Can't Lit: Fearless Fiction from Broken Magazine*. He has a collection of flash fiction called *Fast Fictions*. His poems have been published in *inscribed, 4 and 20 poetry journal*, and *one cool word*. In 2004, he wrote and performed the one-person play *Dislocated Lips* for the Vancouver Fringe Festival. Kevin writes about his schizophrenic father. He is currently completing his MFA in creative writing at the University of British Columbia.

Douglas Todd has received more than fifty journalism honours and fellowships for his features, analyses, news stories, and commentaries. He won the 2005 National Newspaper Award for a first-person piece about his father's battle with schizophrenia. In 2009, he won the top journalism prize from the Canadian Association of University Teachers. He has twice received the Jack Webster Foundation Award for commentary. He is the author of *Brave Souls: Writers and Artists Wrestle with God, Love, Death and the Things That Matter* (Stoddart), and the editor of *Cascadia: The Elusive Utopia—Exploring the Spirit of the Pacific Northwest* (Ronsdale Press, 2008).

Laura Trunkey's short fiction has recently appeared in *Border Crossings, Grain, Fiddlehead*, and in the anthology *Darwin's Bastards: Astounding Tales from Tomorrow* (Douglas & McIntyre, 2010). Her first novel for children, *The Incredibly Ordinary Danny Chandelier* (Annick Press, 2008), was a starred selection on the 2009 Canadian Children's Book Centre's Best Books for Kids and Teens list. A version of "Pennies in My Pocket: Stories of My Brother," recounting the onset of her brother's schizophrenia, was previously published by *Prairie Fire* in 2008 and received two honourable mentions at the National Magazine Awards. She lives in Victoria, British Columbia.

Lynne Van Luven has taught journalism and creative non-fiction at the University of Victoria for the past sixteen years. She has a PHD in Canadian literature with a focus on feminist drama. She is the editor of several anthologies of creative non-fiction: *Going Some Place: Creative Non-Fiction Across Canada* (Coteau Books, 2000), *Nobody's Mother: Life Without Kids* (TouchWood Editions, 2006), *Nobody's Father: Life Without Kids* (TouchWood Editions, 2008) and *Somebody's Child: Stories About Adoption* (TouchWood Editions, 2011), which she co-edited with Bruce Gillespie, and *In the Flesh: Twenty Writers Explore the Body*, which she co-edited with Kathy Page. Lynne writes about her experience with depression in her essay "Life with My Mongrel."

Scott Whyte was born in Portage La Prairie, Manitoba, as the New Year's Baby for 1958. Scott, like his father, joined the Royal Canadian Mounted Police. His father, Assistant Commissioner Dave Whyte, retired from the privilege of commanding the Royal Canadian Mounted Police membership throughout the Province of Alberta and he left with a clean bill of health. Scott was medically discharged with a serious mental illness and a litany of medical irritants, but he has recovered and has forged a new life in California, where he now works as an advocate between the mentally ill and the criminal courts and also provides training on crisis intervention techniques and stress management to law enforcement personnel. Scott writes about post-traumatic stress and bipolar disorder.

Joel Yanofsky is a Montreal writer whose work has appeared in a variety of publications, including *Walrus, Reader's Digest, Canadian Geographic,* and *The Village Voice.* He is a regular book reviewer for *The Montreal Gazette.* His books include *Jacob's Ladder* (Porcupine's Quill), *Homo Erectus: And Other Popular Tales of True Romance* (Signature Editions), and *Mordecai & Me: An Appreciation of a Kind* (Red Deer Press), which won the Mavis Gallant Prize for Nonfiction and the Jewish Book Award. "Bad Day" won *The Malahat Review's* 2008 prize for creative non-fiction as well as a National Magazine Award. The essay also appeared, in somewhat different form, in his memoir, *Bad Animals: A Father's Accidental Education in Autism,* which was published in 2011 by Penguin Canada and won the Mavis Gallant Prize for Non-fiction. It came out in the US from Skyhorse Publishing last spring. His website is joelyanofsky.com.